"At once enormously inspiring and thoroughly pragmatic, this book captivated me from start to finish! It offers an essential road map to help women live better longer with energy, vitality, brain health, and a deep sense of purpose. All women . . . and the men who love them . . . should read this timely book."

—**Marc Freedman,** founder/co-CEO, CoGenerate
(formerly Encore.org), author of *How to Live Forever*

"A comprehensive book on how to create and enjoy an extended health span written by a woman, for women. Expertly researched, easy to understand, and chock-full of practical advice that's also a fun read."

—**Sonia Arrison,** bestselling author of *100+,*
entrepreneur, and investor

"I've spent decades at the forefront of longevity, anti-aging, and sports medicine and welcome this important new book into the timely conversation about how we can positively impact our longevity and wellness with choices that nourish our body, mind, and spirit. *Ageless Aging* shares today's most current thinking and best practices in longevity science to help women take control of their own aging and live their best lives for years to come."

—**Robert Goldman,** MD, world chairman,
International Medical Commission; co-founder and chairman,
World Academy of Anti-Aging Medicine; president emeritus,
National Academy of Sports Medicine

"In *Ageless Aging,* readers will find a nuanced exploration of aging, thoughtfully presented from a woman's perspective. This book takes a deep dive into research findings and expert viewpoints with a keen focus on practical solutions. It offers a thoughtful approach to understanding the complexities of female aging and presents options for those seeking to navigate this stage of life more informed."

—**Jennifer Garrison,** Ph.D., assistant professor,
Buck Institute for Research on Aging

"*Ageless Aging* is a must-read tutorial for anyone interested in maximizing their health, wellness, and joy as well as their longevity as they mature."

—**Mary Furlong,** founder/CEO, Mary Furlong & Associates;
producer of What's Next Longevity Innovation Summit

ALSO BY MADDY DYCHTWALD

Cycles: How We Will Live, Work, and Buy

Influence: How Women's Soaring Economic Power Will Transform Our World for the Better

Gideon's Dream: A Tale of New Beginnings (for children)

Ageless Aging

————————◆————————

A WOMAN'S GUIDE TO INCREASING
HEALTHSPAN, BRAINSPAN, AND LIFESPAN

By Maddy Dychtwald

With Kate Hanley

Mayo Clinic Press

MAYO CLINIC PRESS
200 First St. SW
Rochester, MN 55905
mcpress.mayoclinic.org

MAYO, MAYO CLINIC and the triple-shield Mayo logo are trademarks and
service marks of Mayo Foundation for Medical Education and Research.

The information in this book is true and complete to the best of our knowledge.
This book is intended as an informative guide for those wishing to learn more about
health issues. It is not intended to replace, countermand or conflict with advice
given to you by your own physician. The ultimate decision concerning your care
should be made between you and your doctor. Information in this book is offered
with no guarantees. The author and publisher disclaim all liability in connection
with the use of this book.

The views expressed are the author's personal views, and do not necessarily reflect
the policy or position of Mayo Clinic.

To stay informed about Mayo Clinic Press, please subscribe to our free e-newsletter
at mcpress.mayoclinic.org or follow us on social media.

For bulk sales to employers, member groups and health-related companies, contact
Mayo Clinic at SpecialSalesMayoBooks@mayo.edu.

Proceeds from the sale of every book benefit important medical research and
education at Mayo Clinic.

Cover by Nikolaas Eickelbeck

Library of Congress Control Number: 2023039064

ISBN: 979-8-88770-051-9 hardcover
ISBN: 979-8-88770-052-6 ebook

Printed in Canada

First edition: 2024

To the generations of wonderful women in my family: my mom, Sally, who is no longer with us but is always sitting on my shoulder telling me I can do it; my mother-in-law, Pearl, whose graciousness was a guiding light; and my amazing daughter, Casey, and daughter-in-law, FeyFey, who are both so smart, savvy, kind, and beautiful, inside and out

CONTENTS

Introduction

◆

YOUR LONGEVITY BONUS

Y ou, me, and all of humanity are in the midst of a great leap forward in human longevity. Simply put, we're living much longer than ever before, especially us women . . . and we're not necessarily well prepared for this journey of longer life.

Up until about the turn of the twentieth century, most people didn't age, they died. Sure, some people lived long lives, but they were the exception, not the rule. On the first day of the twentieth century, January 1, 1900, the average American lived to age forty-seven. By the end of that century, average American life expectancy had skyrocketed to seventy-nine years, more than an extra three decades of life. The COVID-19 pandemic took a bite out of this—about two years—but longevity is projected to rise by another five to ten years in the next decade or two. And with numerous breakthroughs in medicine, technology, and research that have the potential to prevent or reverse disease on the horizon, that number is sure to go up even more than projected. Incredibly, centenarians are now the fastest-growing segment of the world's population.

This news is even more meaningful for women, because we live an average of six years longer than men. I call these extra years our *longevity bonus*. It's a little like we've won the longevity lottery. In fact, a full 80 percent of the centenarians alive today are women. It is entirely feasible that you may live to one hundred.

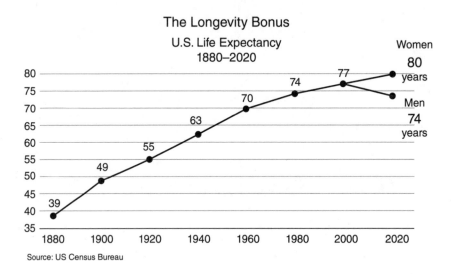

The Longevity Bonus

U.S. Life Expectancy
1880–2020

Source: US Census Bureau

But there's a downside to this bonus, and it's no joke: as Judith Lorber and Lisa Jean Moore point out in their book *Gendered Bodies: Feminist Perspectives*, men die quicker, but women get sicker. Our healthspans—the number of years we live in good health and vitality—don't match our lifespans. Women tend to spend more years in poor health at the end of their lives than men do, even when you correct for their longer lives.

The net result is that millions of women spend the last years of life coping with aches and pains and undergoing an increasing number of treatments for chronic degenerative diseases such as cancer, heart disease, and diabetes. And even before we reach our final years, we spend a lot of time and energy worrying about eventually outliving our money and being a burden to our families.

Unfortunately, this is how I started to feel when I was in my sixties. I developed terrible pain in my hips, and eventually it got so bad that, after decades of an active and healthy lifestyle, I was walking with a limp, which made me feel older than my chronological age. I struggled to come up with any real solutions for my pain. I got by on over-the-counter anti-inflammatories, but I knew that wasn't a long-term strategy. I experimented with massage, acupuncture, platelet-rich plasma (PRP) treatments, and pretty much everything legal except opioids, but any relief was short-lived.

My mind went to dark places, imagining all the experiences I would miss in my later years—traveling with my family, taking a rigorous hike with friends, and playing on the floor with my grandkids (even though they were just an idea at that point—and still are).

Finally, in desperation, I had an MRI. It revealed a scary picture. Due to genetic hip dysplasia (which I was unaware of), I had worn down the cartilage to the point that I was literally bone-on-bone in both hips. With every movement, the bones were rubbing against each other, causing friction, more damage, and excruciating pain. Even the surgeons were surprised to see such an extreme case in someone of my age. (I was sixty-eight when I first learned this—youngish for this to take place.)

I went from doctor to doctor, trying to figure out the right action for me. Finally I asked a top orthopedic surgeon specializing in hip surgery at the University of California, San Francisco (UCSF), what he would do if he were me. He said, "I'd do both hips at once through an anterior procedure. And I'd have it done by a surgeon who does nothing but hip surgeries and specializes in bilateral replacement." I took his advice, but the surgeon I found had a three-month waiting list. What was I supposed to do in the meantime?

When I asked my orthopedist for advice on *precovery*—things I could do to manage pain, keep my life going, and prepare for a successful surgery and recovery—he told me to buy a cane. I thought he was kidding, but he was not.

I was convinced there had to be a better solution. So I doubled down on yoga and Pilates to further strengthen my core. After some digging, I learned that inflammation was worsening my pain. I sought advice from several experts such as Dr. Mark Hyman, at the Cleveland Clinic, and Rudi Tanzi, PhD, at Harvard University, who recommended that I try an anti-inflammatory diet. Although many in the traditional medical community dismissed this type of diet as mere hype or as too difficult to follow, I was willing to try anything. I cut out dairy, gluten, and most sugar (an anti-inflammatory way of eating that is now increasingly recommended for lifelong brain health). In truth, the only thing I didn't cut out was wine; let's be honest, it just feels good to have an occasional glass of wine at the end of the day.

What may sound like a sad way to live—forgoing all those types of foods—resulted in a huge win: within six weeks, *all* of the pain in my hips went away. I got my life back! I even considered not doing the surgery, but bone-on-bone isn't a good foundation for long-term health.

I didn't stop there. I continued to build my precovery plan. As I dug deeper, I discovered the work of pioneering experts like Peggy Huddleston, a psychotherapist and researcher who does mindfulness training at Brigham and Women's Hospital in Boston. She showed me how meditation, affirmations, and my network of friends and family could optimize my resilience and speed my recovery. It helped drive home the point that the body, mind, and spirit are intimately interconnected—both in sickness and in health.

When I finally had the double hip surgery, my recovery was remarkable. I was in the hospital for only one night, despite being told it would be at least three. I was walking—including navigating stairs—without a cane or walker within a few days, though I'd been warned that it would be at least a few weeks before that happened. And I was fully recovered and back to my normal activities within a month. (Of course, this is my individual experience, and for many people, even with all the precovery in the world, this may not be the outcome.)

This is just one example of our body's ability to bounce back from trauma and disease—and even recover from physical and mental deterioration linked with aging.

Now, as I write this at seventy-three, I feel stronger and more resilient than I did at sixty-eight, or even at fifty-eight. While I still primarily eat an anti-inflammatory diet, that doesn't mean I don't indulge in pizza and ice cream. I do, but I definitely feel a little more achy in my joints and a little less clear in my mind when I do, both of which are good reminders to get right back to the eating pattern that I know works best for me.

The experience reinforced what I already knew—you don't get to your seventies without experiencing some real shit. I'm guessing you may have already noticed that, too. The good news is that all the things you do to make the most of your longevity bonus make you more resilient, no matter what life throws your way.

WHY I WROTE THIS BOOK

I'm not only a woman facing her own aging; I'm also close to a forty-year veteran of the fields of aging and longevity. In 1986, my husband, Ken, and I founded Age Wave, long considered North America's leading think tank and consultancy on aging, longevity, and retirement issues. While I am not a doctor, a financial advisor, or a spiritual guru (and you should of course consult with your doctor about any health concerns you have and your financial advisor about investment strategies), I am a thought leader, writer, researcher, social scientist, and longtime curator of information about longevity and aging in the areas of health, mental and emotional well-being, retirement, lifestyle, and finances. As a direct result of my work and my personal experience, I strongly believe women should be leading this longevity revolution, especially since we are the ones who are typically living longer. I also believe that the more informed we are, the more proactive we can be about making the choices and taking the actions that can foster better health in all areas of our lives.

Over the years at Age Wave, we've completed landmark research (albeit not medical research) with more than 200,000 survey respondents, conducted countless focus groups worldwide, interviewed other top experts, and analyzed thousands of reports, papers, and datasets.

My work at Age Wave gives me direct access to top researchers and academics in a wide swath of fields (including medicine, psychology, and gerontology), clinicians, and financial professionals. In this book, I'll share not only what they recommend to their patients and clients, but also what they are doing for themselves and what they whisper in the ears of the women they care about: their personal recipes for extending both healthspan and lifespan.

Throughout this book I recommend certain products or services to help you implement the information included on these pages and that I either use myself or have researched. I don't benefit in any way from the sales of these products.

WHY YOU NEED TO READ THIS BOOK

It's time for us women to learn how to better match our healthspan to our lifespan so that our longer life is a gift, not a curse. We women can show the world how long life can be done right and what can be accomplished with all these extra years. To do this, women need to be at the center of the conversation, shaping the future of longevity. Women hold the power to change the narrative of longevity and aging for all—to emphasize the gifts of long life while taking the steps needed to prevent, delay, and minimize physical and mental deterioration. These common effects of aging are the biggest downsides of long life, and they keep us from seeing the full upside of longevity—including our wisdom, experience, resilience, and perspective.

How can we make the most of our longevity bonus and model a healthier, more vital aging, exactly?

In these pages, you'll learn—and, more importantly, *own*—the truth that, to a great extent, you can heavily influence your healthspan, your brainspan, and maybe even your lifespan.

You'll be able to customize a holistic recipe to guide your aging journey. Going well beyond the basics, the approach I outline on these pages acknowledges the interconnection between our body, mind, and spirit; our health and sense of purpose; and our financial well-being and mental and physical health. After all, the different facets of your life don't exist in separate silos. If you aren't moving your body much, your mental health and sleep can suffer. If you're sleep deprived, your appetite and your hormones can get out of whack. If you are worried about money, it can negatively impact your physical and mental health. The positive reframing of these truths is that when you start taking care of one aspect of your life, others are likely to improve as well—a rising tide that lifts all boats.

HOW TO USE THIS BOOK

You can begin to reap the benefits of this approach in a matter of weeks. Those quick wins can motivate you to keep moving forward, taking more steps toward expanding your healthspan and maybe even your lifespan. In each chapter, I've included practical tips, techniques, and hacks that I've categorized according to level of experience. Many of these are free and easy to implement. I also include an "if you do one thing" feature so that you'll know the simplest and most impactful step to get you started.

I recognize that creating and continuing to add new habits and patterns is challenging. I provide guidance on how to customize your action plan to what's feasible for you now—and how to build on it as you go. The good news is that the change you can experience from tending to these areas of your life isn't incremental, it's exponential. That means each change you make will give you more energy and inspiration to make another change, and another. After all, the greater the number of thoughtfully chosen elements you add to your recipe, the richer, more satisfying your finished dish is going to be.

Wherever you are in your aging journey, it's never too late to invest in your well-being, or to reinvent yourself. It is possible for life to get better and better as you age, especially when you are open to the idea that our longevity bonus can be an ascent, not a decline. Let's take off, together.

Part 1

⸻ ◆ ⸻

THE NEW LONGEVITY

1

SIPPING FROM THE FOUNTAIN OF YOUTHFULNESS

I coined the term *ageless aging* in the 1990s when I was a guest speaker at the Golden Door spa for a group of highly successful women executives on a retreat to help them de-stress and think about their future in out-of-the-box ways. Back then, fifty and sixty were considered over the hill, especially for women. I wanted these women to know that it doesn't have to be that way. And now I'm saying the same thing to you.

What exactly do I mean by *ageless aging*? If you open the dictionary to find the definition of *ageless*, the first word to appear is *timeless*. While you can't stop the Earth from turning and time from passing, you *can* minimize the negative effects of the passage of time and choose to not let your chronological age and the stereotypes around aging limit you or the choices you make. With knowledge, action, and a little bit of luck, you may maximize the upsides of longevity while minimizing or even avoiding many of the downsides that we've come to accept as inevitable—losing your memory, your mobility, your health, and your joy for life.

No matter how old you are, there is still a lot of life to be lived. Making the most of your remaining years requires you to prepare yourself for the journey physically, mentally, emotionally, and spiritually. Taking advantage of the latest cutting-edge scientific breakthroughs in longevity can help, too—especially those that apply specifically to women.

I think of it like this: When I was in my twenties and trying to make it as a working actor in Los Angeles, I succumbed to the toxic fear of aging that was rampant in Hollywood (and still is) and splurged on a fancy facial in a dermatologist's office. As the nurse practitioner worked her magic, she said something that really stuck with me: *People are like high-performance cars—you need to feed yourself the right fuel, get the maintenance you need, and have regular checkups so you don't end up in the junkyard.*

I didn't love thinking of myself as a car, but I saw the logic in what she was saying. You can't ignore the many forms of routine maintenance that vehicles require and still expect your car to run well—or even at all—for decades to come. Yes, Fords, Hondas, and Subarus are all built to run for multiple hundreds of thousands of miles, but not if you don't change the oil, rotate the tires, and replace the filters and belts and whatever else they do at those regularly scheduled service appointments. And the same is true for you. You can't expect to be dynamic, vibrant, and healthy well into your eighties, nineties, and beyond without doing the things a body—especially a female body— needs to perform its best.

I just want to say right up front that I am 100 percent nonjudgmental about what you or anyone else chooses to do in the name of aging agelessly. I have friends who have had all manner of lifts and tucks who look fabulous, and I applaud them (and sometimes covet their results). There is definitely a spectrum when it comes to how to embrace the outward signs of your longevity. Some women proudly flaunt their gray hair and wrinkles as a welcome sign of their elder status, and I applaud them. Others choose to tweak the physical signs of aging by dyeing their hair and pursuing natural and/or surgical treatments they can afford and feel comfortable doing. That's fine, too. Wherever you fall on that spectrum, you are welcome here. But that's just the external, *appearance* side of the ageless aging equation. This book is focused not so much on physical appearance as on increasing your healthspan, brainspan, and maybe even lifespan. By doing that, your physical appearance is bound to improve as well. The truth is, if you want to enjoy your longevity bonus, you can't just hope for the best or trust that you'll find a silver-bullet supplement, medication, or aesthetic treatment. There are just too many potholes in the road of life, especially for women fifty and over. Ageless aging is much more than skin-deep—and, frankly, it's more life-enhancing.

PREPARING FOR THE ROAD AHEAD

I bet that as a woman in your forties, fifties, sixties, or seventies, you've experienced a lightbulb moment when you realized that your life is far from over. Perhaps it's because you've been paying attention to the media reporting around longevity. Or because now that you've arrived at your current age, you realize that you are nowhere near "old" in the traditional sense of the word.

Sure, you may wonder if you'll have the necessary physical, mental, emotional, spiritual, and financial resilience and vitality to meet whatever challenges lie ahead. And you probably have moments of fear of declining health or dwindling money (worries that are justified; more on those in a moment). But now that you've gotten to this point in your life—and maybe it's coinciding with your kids leaving home, or some other kind of ending or new beginning, whether it's a job or a relationship—you can see that you've got time. Not just time to fill with hobbies, although hobbies are great, but time to fulfill your existing dreams or even dream up new ones.

The truth is, given our expanding lifespans, it's possible that you could live into your eighties or nineties, or even past one hundred. Even if you're well into midlife, you could still have *decades* left.

As exciting as that possibility is, it's also more than a little scary. It may leave you asking questions like:

- What foods, supplements, exercise, health hacks, and personal relationships can boost my overall immunity and resilience?
- What steps can I take now to keep my brain functioning at its highest levels and perhaps even prevent (or at least delay) dementia?
- How do I prepare to deal with the unforeseen situations life might throw my way, like health issues, losing a spouse or loved one, or being a caregiver for a loved one?
- How can I avoid being a burden on my family and loved ones?
- How do I make sure I have financial peace of mind throughout a long life?
- How do I discover (or rediscover) a sense of purpose to make the most of the years in front of me?

WOMEN AND LONGEVITY

One of the big stories of our time is that we're at the dawn of a longevity revolution that has never happened before. What's more, women are leading the way, living an average of six years longer than men. (The estrogen our body makes is thought to be the key, as it promotes the expression of longevity-associated genes and the creation of antioxidant enzymes that can then protect against the harmful effects of inflammation—although, of course, we lose this protection after menopause.) But as I touched on briefly in the introduction, that perk has a major downside: according to an analysis of data from the World Health Organization's Global Health Observatory, the average woman in the United States will spend the last twelve years of her life in a cascade of poor health. This combination of longer lifespan but poorer healthspan is what is now generally referred to as the *gender and health paradox*.[1]

In other words, our healthspans and lifespans are out of sync. As you can imagine, this means you may be more limited in the activities you take part in. Your healthcare costs may go up, too, which means that your money—which already has to last longer than men's, owing to our longer lives—gets even more stretched.

This raises another question: since women live longer than men, why is so much of the conversation around longevity being led by men? It's high time we women own the topic and become longevity pioneers, leading the way to ageless aging. Living a long life is a privilege that many people never get the opportunity to enjoy. Those of us who do get the opportunity should embrace it and rewrite the script.

One of the most powerful places to start is by changing our own attitudes toward living longer and growing older.

AGEISM IS HIDING IN PLAIN SIGHT

Another threat to healthspan has to do with our attitudes regarding an -ism that doesn't get the attention it deserves: ageism, or the view that older people are somehow "less than" younger people—less vital, less smart, less able, less valued. Social entrepreneur Marc Freedman recently described ageism to me in a way that really put it aptly—and bluntly: "age apartheid."

Most of us—often subconsciously—have internalized stereotypes about what it means to be "old." There are a lot of negative presumptions, especially for women. Research shows that our society tends to view mature women as "old" at a younger age than men, and to frame that negatively, whereas men—particularly in the workplace—are often seen as more influential and powerful the older they become.[2]

To a great extent, ageism is programmed by popular culture. And even though we have made big strides in representation for different races, sexual orientations, gender identities, and physical abilities, older people remain woefully underrepresented. It may be the last accepted -ism. According to Nadia Tuma-Weldon, EVP, global head of thought leadership at McCann Worldgroup and executive vice president of the agency's global intelligence unit, Truth Central, "Age is the last frontier that we don't talk about. In fact, it is still okay to ignore or even make fun of older people." As one example, clothing companies have started using models who represent all body types and skin tones. However, the one constant that remains is that they are mostly all young.

Oprah Winfrey, sixty-nine years old at this writing, describes it like this: "We live in a youth-obsessed culture that is constantly trying to tell us that if we are not young, and we're not glowing, and we're not hot, that we don't matter." Dr. Imani Woody, a nationally recognized thought leader on aging, describes it as *erasure* and says it's worse than what she has experienced as a Black woman and a lesbian. These can be serious headwinds.

There's no doubt that our culture is still biased toward youth, which greatly contributes to our fears of getting older and, ultimately, our prejudice against aging. Don't get me wrong: there are wonderful things about being young. And as with everything else, there are also some downsides—impulsivity, a lack of self-knowledge and self-awareness, and difficulty putting things in perspective chief among them.

Although our culture absolutely shapes our views on growing older, each of us helps perpetuate ageism both in the world at large and in our own minds. If you've ever said "I just had a senior moment," or "I'm too old to change my ways," or "You can't teach an old dog new tricks," you've associated being older with being somehow impaired. And if you've ever looked in the mirror and shuddered at a gray hair, a wrinkle, or sagging skin, well, there's another way your fear of growing older and negative thoughts about age are showing up.

I admit, I participate in ageism, too. Every time I give a presentation, I tell the crowd how old I am. I do it to show that this is what seventy-three can be like; it can be feeling vital and energetic, doing important work, and pursuing purpose. But I am playing into the ageist perception of what a woman my age is stereotypically supposed to look like and be like. Ageism is so ingrained in us, and in many ways it is still hidden in plain sight.

That's not to say it's bad to share how old you are with others. When I spoke with Ashton Applewhite, pro-aging activist and author of *This Chair Rocks: A Manifesto Against Ageism*, she told me, "It's important to claim your age and in the same breath push back against the fixed meanings that our culture attaches to that number." But every one of us will have our own realities and comfort levels that we have to understand. Applewhite shared with me a story about a talk on ageism she was giving in the early 2010s to a group of women in Beverly Hills. "I suggested that we have everyone who has a question say how old they are. And the organizer of the event said, 'Honey, this is Beverly Hills. We would need ambulances.'" When Applewhite laughed, the event organizer replied, "You don't get it. If I didn't dye my hair, I would lose my job, and I have children to support."

Applewhite added, "Ever since then I qualify my remarks more carefully. We each, especially as women, need to negotiate this stuff in our own way, at our own speed, and judge each other last."

HOW OLD DO YOU THINK YOU ARE?

Popular myths and stereotypes about our worth and value decreasing as we get older are just that: myths and stereotypes. We women are not destined to become vulnerable, frail, and sick as we age, nor are we destined to become socially isolated and irrelevant. We have to believe these truths ourselves first.

Dolly Parton once said, "I don't think about my life in terms of numbers. I ain't never gonna be old, because I ain't got time to be old." Research has shown that our preconceived, stereotyped notions of chronological age can dictate how we age—even how old we look, feel, and behave—which makes many of us (like Dolly) feel boxed in.

Yale gerontologist Becca Levy, PhD, has conducted considerable research into the effects of preconceptions about age on health outcomes, and her findings are nothing short of astonishing. Perhaps the most jaw-dropping is a finding from her 2002 research that followed hundreds of people over age fifty in a small Ohio town for two decades: those who had a positive view of aging had a median survival rate that was 7.5 years longer than those who saw it through a negative lens. According to Levy, "The single most important factor in determining longevity—more important than gender, income, social background, loneliness or functional health—is how people think about and approach the idea of old age."[3]

Levy's research shows that viewing the aging process and capabilities of older people—including yourself—positively can help ward off many of the things we tend to fear the most about living a long time. It halves the risk of cardiovascular events (such as heart failure, heart attack, and stroke),[4] helps ward off mental illnesses such as depression and anxiety,[5] encourages a quicker recovery from bouts of disability,[6] and even reduces the risk of developing Alzheimer's.[7] Best of all, her research shows that it's never too late to amend your views of aging to become more positive.

If you're now wondering whether you might be harboring some negative ideas about aging, Levy has created a short online quiz that's helpful in revealing your thoughts on older people. Visit it at https://becca-levy.com/quiz to assess how positive or negative your views of aging are compared to other people who have taken the quiz.

It's not just Levy and her team of researchers who are uncovering the power of how we think to positively—or negatively—affect our healthspan and lifespan. The nascent field of geroscience is now revealing that there are more factors within your control that influence how you age. For instance, "age identity," or what chronological age you identify with no matter how many years you've lived, has an effect.

When Korean researchers did MRI scans of women and men over forty, they found that the brains of those with a lower age identity had significantly more gray matter in their brain compared to others whose subjective age matched their chronological age.[8] (Gray matter makes up the outermost layer of the brain and is associated with perception, processing sensations, and the ability to think and reason—it also plays a role in memory. Gray matter often shrinks in those with Alzheimer's disease.)

In other words, your body is impacted by how old you think and feel you are. Perhaps it's time that we stopped thinking of our age as an absolute. Just as we have had a cultural awakening around gender—recognizing that something that we long considered to be biologically fixed is a social construct—maybe we can start acknowledging that chronological age is, too. Just as Facebook has restructured its gender dropdown menu so that users get to choose from fifty-two different gender identities, perhaps soon we'll be able to select from options such as "I'm fifty-six but feel thirty-five" on our social media profiles. It's not as far-fetched as it sounds: Emile Ratelband, a Dutch politician, TV personality, and life coach, felt there were such vast gaps between his chronological age, biological age, and psychological age that, in 2018, when he was sixty-nine years old, he (unsuccessfully) petitioned the courts to lower his age by twenty years. In an interview with the *Washington Post*, Ratelband explained, "We can make our own decisions if we want to change our name or even our gender. My feelings about my mind and body is that I'm about 40 or 45." Yes, I wish this was an example of a woman, but you get the point: the passage of time is inevitable, but how we evolve physically, mentally, and emotionally does not have to follow the same trajectory as that of time.

It's one thing to understand that the foods you eat and exercises you do can help you age more agelessly, but it's quite another to understand that your attitudes about aging itself and how old you *feel* have such an enormous impact on your physical health. The takeaway is that we have more control over how we age—with more tools to help us exert that influence—than ever before.

One of the best starting places for influencing your ageless aging is to shift your own bias away from the refrain that fifty or sixty or even seventy is over the hill, and to stop telling yourself that you're "too old" for anything.

While researching this book I've had the pleasure and the privilege of talking to many women who are making the most of their longevity bonus, and DeEtte Sauer is at the top of the list. DeEtte was a child of alcoholics who grew up as part of the Cajun culture in Baton Rouge, Louisiana, where drinking, smoking, eating, and letting the good times roll (or *laissez les bon temps rouler*, as they say in Louisiana) were a way of life. She and her husband were both addicted to alcohol before finally quitting—and essentially replacing that addiction with one to cigarettes and nicotine. In her forties, DeEtte smoked her last cigarette, and once again transferred her addiction. (She also lost her oldest daughter to a car accident—certainly enough to drive anyone to want to numb out.) This time, her addiction was eating. "I quit drinking at thirty-nine and then I blew up until I was forty-six," DeEtte told me. "I love to cook, but I made all the wrong foods." Her church didn't help. "The potluck suppers and the donuts in the morning before church made eating unhealthy foods perfectly acceptable." Finally, DeEtte's husband told her that he was no longer attracted to her. "This is a gentle man who has just adored me from the beginning. It shattered me."

It shattered her, and then it inspired her. DeEtte went back to school to study food and alcohol counseling, and then used those tools to address her own addiction. She started reading everything she could about health, including Dan Buettner's work on Blue Zones—the areas of the world where the most centenarians live. She went to work for a hospital teaching weight management.

From there, DeEtte added in more exercise—starting a walking group with friends in her neighborhood, and then, when that helped her have more energy, going to the gym with her husband. (Yes, they stayed married after that comment, although they did separate for a couple of months right after it.) For several years she focused on the bike and the treadmill, but then DeEtte's gym posted a flyer that they were starting a swimming team. DeEtte thought, "Maybe swimming is the sport I could compete in." The only problem? No, it was not that she was fifty-eight at the time. It was that she couldn't swim.

That first morning practice, "I was humiliated because everybody else was ten or fifteen years younger, and I couldn't even swim across the pool." DeEtte tried to tell the twenty-two-year-old coach that she'd made a mistake, but the coach wasn't having it. "She just got right in my face, and she said, 'Keep your mouth shut and do what I tell you. You're strong and I'm going to teach you.' And she did."

After swimming for about three months, DeEtte entered her first meet. She lost, but she also recorded her fastest time ever. "I was going 'Yay, yay, yay,' when the woman who beat me said, 'Why are you happy? You were so slow.'" DeEtte used that woman's remarks to motivate her. You'll be happy to know that DeEtte went on to beat that other woman many times—and that she has also medaled in the Senior Games multiple times since.

It may sound like a lot of effort and discipline and you may wonder if you have it, but for DeEtte, it's really about finding her bliss. That's right: her bliss.

DeEtte has so much fun swimming that she describes her morning swim practices as "a play date before you do your life." She went on to say, "We're giggling and laughing and cutting up like kids." The energy she gets from swimming—the community, the sense of achievement, and the physical fitness—fuels her volunteer work, teaching disadvantaged kids to read.

DeEtte's upward spiral all started with eating healthier. One change opened the door to the next. To the point that now, decades later, she says, "My eightieth year was the best year I've ever had—I swam at the Senior Games, where there were twelve thousand athletes in all the different sports. And I won more gold medals than any other person there. I've never been so happy in all my life."

If DeEtte had stayed on the path she was on in her thirties and early forties, she likely would never have made it to her eighties, much less become a world-class athlete engaged in so many varied activities in her life. It wasn't too late for her to make changes that helped her age agelessly, and hopefully it's not too late for you, either.

THE SCIENCE OF AGING

Aging is a lifelong process that begins in the womb and continues until we die. Certain predictable changes happen at the cellular and molecular levels as humans live longer. These hallmarks of aging not only help us understand why we become more prone to chronic disease the older we get, but also point toward ways we can positively influence the aging process itself. Using the hallmarks of aging as a guide, scientists are now looking for cures for age-related conditions and even, according to many longevity experts, a potential cure for aging itself. (Yes, there is a group of scientists and thought leaders who think of aging itself as a disease to be cured.)

When I spoke with James Kirkland, MD, PhD, director of the Center of Aging at Mayo Clinic, he explained that the hallmarks can be influenced positively. Better yet, he said, "We've found that when you target one [hallmark of aging], you tend to affect all the rest."

For those of you who, like me, want to understand the science of what's going on in their own bodies, here's a nutshell description of the hallmarks of aging that longevity experts are looking to positively impact:

- **Cellular senescence.** One of the hallmarks of aging that we have long known about is senescent cells—cells that have stopped dividing but don't die. They are normally swept away by the immune system, but this removal does not keep up with new senescent cell generation that occurs with aging and in a number of diseases. While some level of senescent cells is normal and even beneficial (researchers theorize that senescent cells are what produce the factors that trigger labor in pregnant women), when they accumulate and persist—as often happens with living longer—they contribute to inflammation and most of the other pillars of aging that follow.

- **Shortening or dysfunctional telomeres.** In 1982, Elizabeth Blackburn at UCSF and Jack Szostak at Harvard discovered telomeres, which are specialized structures made of genetic material and proteins that are found at the ends of our chromosomes. They're like the plastic tips on your shoelaces. Every time a cell divides, the telomeres get a little shorter. Once telomeres get short or dysfunctional enough, that cell will stop dividing and will die or become senescent.

- **DNA damage.** Your genetic material incurs damage thanks to the byproducts of normal cellular processes and environmental influences (such as radiation exposure from flying in airplanes or heavy metals ingested in food or supplements).

- **Epigenetic dysregulation.** There are a multitude of chemical compounds and proteins that attach to your DNA—known as your epigenome—which dictate whether a gene is turned on or turned off. As you age, epigenetic shifts tend to turn on more bad genes, such as those that promote inflammation, and turn off more good genes, such as those that suppress tumors.

- **Mitochondrial decline.** Your mitochondria are organelles located within your cells that produce the energy needed to fuel the myriad functions of your body. Over time, these energy factories lose efficiency.

- **Stem cell depletion.** Stem cells play an important role in repairing and replenishing the body. As we age, they decline in quantity and can mutate, impairing their function.

- **Glycation.** This is what happens when a sugar molecule bonds with a protein or a fat, and the end result—known as a glycation end product—can accumulate as you grow older, contributing to wrinkles, cataracts, atherosclerosis, and Alzheimer's (this speaks to why it's so important to be super mindful about your sugar consumption).

- **Other cellular processes**—including intracellular communication, nutrient sensing, and maintaining the right balance of proteins within cells—decline in a predictable way with age.

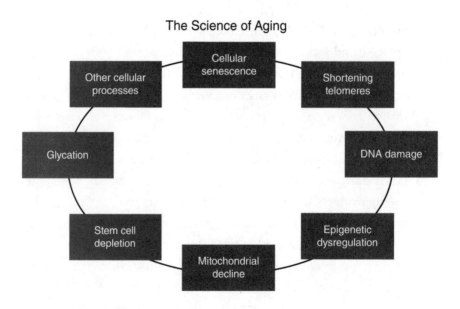

The Science of Aging

As you can see, the physical aspect of aging is no joke. I'm sharing these things that science has labeled the hallmarks of aging so that you can see what you're up against—you can't simply hope that aging won't catch up with you. *How* you can positively influence these processes is what we'll dive into throughout the rest of this book.

Three Kinds of Aging

To really embrace all the things ageless aging can be, it's important to understand the three kinds of aging.

Chronological aging is the most obvious form of aging and the one that remains indifferent to our whims, desires, and discoveries. It is dependent only on the passing of time. Every day, we become a day older. We are not alone: the same is true for trees, frogs, and even the sun. Simple.

Psychological aging is the normal emotional developmental process of maturing as a result of the various experiences of our lives. Throughout this sometimes easy, sometimes bumpy process, we continually redefine and renegotiate our beliefs, priorities, and motivating passions and, in the process, develop psychological benefits such as resilience, perspective, confidence, knowledge, and maybe even wisdom.

In regard to the overall context of aging, psychological aging is usually thought of as a positive experience, and those people who are most psychologically mature are thought of as being "wise." It usually comes as a great compliment when one is told that she or he is an enlightened "old soul."

Physical aging or **biological aging** is probably the one kind of aging that no one looks forward to (at least, not once we pass those ages that open up new freedoms, like being able to drive a car at sixteen or purchase alcohol at twenty-one). Most of us think of the physical aging journey as one of loss—loss of health, sexual potency, fertility, beauty, coordination, strength, value, and vitality. Since these are qualities that most of us treasure and enjoy, it makes sense that the idea of losing these attributes frightens and troubles us.

Physical or biological aging is also a measure of your body's ability to function, and it is influenced greatly by your diet, exercise, and other lifestyle choices. You could be age fifty-four chronologically but have a biological age that is younger, about the same, or older than the number of years you've been alive.

Slowing down or even reversing your biological aging process is an essential part of ageless aging—it's decoupling your chronological age from your overall physical health. It's extending your healthspan to better match your lifespan so that you have the energy, passion, and vitality to make the most of your longevity bonus. For instance, when I tested my biological age (using a test that analyzed my epigenetics), my biological age was fifty-two. At the time of testing, I was chronologically seventy-one. Needless to say, I felt gratified that all the steps I've taken to age more agelessly seem to be having a positive impact. If I can do it, so can you!

TAKE CONTROL OF YOUR HALLMARKS OF AGING

Today, thanks to rapidly growing interest in the subject, scientists, doctors, and research institutions increasingly view aging as malleable, something that can be impacted, slowed down, and maybe even reversed. For instance, we've known for decades that calorie restriction appears to extend life and delay biological aging (the first animal study to document the link was published in 1935). Then in the 1990s, UCSF microbiologist Cynthia Kenyon upended the idea that aging was an unavoidable, irreversible process when she discovered that a single genetic mutation could significantly expand lifespan in worms, and the race was on to develop products to fight aging and the diseases and conditions that can occur as we live longer.

Kenyon's groundbreaking work has led to a flurry of longevity research worldwide. According to Longevity Fund founder Laura Deming, researchers are "trying to figure out what kinds of damage accumulates with age, how to reverse that accumulation, and then search for the switches we can flip in human biology to increase lifespan." I would add that, even more important, researchers are discovering ways to increase our healthspan, and many of the tips, techniques, and practices that they have so far uncovered are what I'll share throughout this book.

GOODBYE (AND GOOD RIDDANCE) TO THE 70/30 RULE

When viewed through the lens of the hallmarks of aging, physical aging is a complex process of things just wearing out. We now know that each of us can affect the pace at which our own wearing out happens. Prior to Cynthia Kenyon's work, the common assumption in both science and medicine was that, while lifestyle certainly played a role in health and aging, it was greatly outweighed by genetics. That was the original 70/30 rule: 70 percent of aging and longevity was determined by genetics, and just 30 percent was based on lifestyle and environment.

In 1998 that assumption was flipped on its head once and for all by key findings of the MacArthur Foundation Research Network on Successful Aging (an initiative that brings together a multidisciplinary team of researchers from a variety of institutions to study the most pressing challenges of our time), which asserted that 70 percent of our health and longevity is firmly under our control, based on lifestyle and environment, and only 30 percent is controlled by our genes. As Dr. John W. Rowe, director of the MacArthur Foundation aging initiative and founding director of the Division on Aging at Harvard Medical School, puts it, "People are largely responsible for how they age."

Since then, we've realized that's even *more* true than initially suggested, as scientists have proposed that the ratio is actually closer to 80/20 in favor of lifestyle and environment. And that ratio has just been refined even further: Google's Calico Labs, a biotech firm focused on researching the biology that controls aging and lifespan with the hope of discovering and developing interventions that enable people to live longer and healthier lives, recently asserted that 90 percent of our health and longevity is controlled by our lifestyle and environment and only 10 percent by our genetics. I'll take that math any day.

There's no question this is a game changer. Lifestyle management has emerged as *the* most potent tool in our ageless aging toolbox. Of course, it isn't a new idea—we've been hearing "Move it or lose it" and "You are what you eat" for years. The difference is that today we have a swiftly growing body of scientific evidence and data to underscore exactly how important these choices are, and which ones produce the very best results.

From what we understand at this point, the true power of lifestyle comes from epigenetics, which determines which genes get expressed and which don't. And the choices you make every day affect your epigenetics. I spoke to Dr. Stephen Kopecky, a cardiologist at Mayo Clinic, author of *Live Younger Longer*, and a huge proponent of prevention, who explained it this way: "It turns out that good lifestyle turns on good genes and turns off bad genes. And so, even people with bad genes can lower their risk of having heart attacks and dying early by 75 to 80 percent." Your lifestyle can't change your predisposition toward disease; that's in your genes. But it can certainly lower your risk; that's epigenetics. So now let's take a look at how your lifestyle choices are affecting your risk.

AGELESS AGING SELF-ASSESSMENT

When it comes to maximizing how you age, it boils down to not only understanding the small- and large-scale decisions you can make, but also putting them into action. It's that second step that so many women struggle with. I call this the *intention/action gap*. Let me explain. In a 2020 Age Wave study, we learned that most women have a strong understanding of lifestyle changes that can increase their healthspan, but they don't always put that information into action. We found that 93 percent of women fifty and over understood the basics of what to do to stay healthy longer, yet only 53 percent of them actually do it. It's not just what you know (or will learn in this book); it's taking action that really matters.

I find one of the most powerful ways to get me motivated to take action and start building new habits and attitudes is to do a clear assessment of what I'm currently doing and not doing. I designed this simple assessment with input from experts and nationally recognized guidelines to help you quickly see how many things you are doing that could be eroding your healthspan, what I have labeled "age accelerants," as well as how many things you're doing that can help extend it, what I'm calling "age decelerants."

To assess your current efforts to age more agelessly and expand your healthspan to better match your lifespan, put a check mark alongside every element you do regularly. Be honest! And use a pencil—you can come back and take this assessment again once you've worked through the rest of this book and see how many checkmarks have moved from the "age accelerant" to the "age decelerant" column. Taking stock of where you are now will help you measure your progress once you've added more health-promoting ingredients to your recipe.

Step one: Put a check mark (in pencil) next to each item that you do regularly.

Age Accelerants	Age Decelerants
☐ Sleep less than 7 hours	☐ Allow for at least 7 hours of sleep
☐ Regularly awaken two or more times a night	☐ Regularly feel you've slept soundly
☐ Go a day (or more) without exercising	☐ Get 30 minutes of moderate exercise at least 5 times a week
☐ Smoke or vape	☐ Lift weights regularly
☐ Drink more than one alcoholic drink a day	☐ Have a regular mindfulness practice (like meditating, doing yoga or tai chi, or praying)
☐ Sit more than three hours without getting up	☐ Stand or get up out of your seat every hour or so

Age Accelerants	Age Decelerants
☐ Skip brushing teeth	☐ Brush and floss
☐ Eat sweets (cookies, pie, ice cream, candy)	☐ Stick to fruit and/or dark chocolate to satisfy sweet tooth
☐ Eat fried or charred foods	☐ Avoid fried or charred foods
☐ Go a whole day without eating a fresh fruit or vegetable	☐ Eat leafy greens, cruciferous veg, or deeply hued vegetables daily
☐ Eat ultra-processed foods	☐ Eat primarily whole foods
☐ Drink soda or fruit juice	☐ Drink half your body weight (in ounces) of water daily
☐ Drink sweet coffee drinks or sweet tea	☐ Drink unsweetened coffee or tea
☐ Eat processed meats such as sausage, bacon, and hot dogs	☐ Eat fatty fish such as salmon
☐ Eat right before bedtime	☐ Eat fermented foods
☐ Stay on screens right up until bedtime	☐ Spend at least 30 minutes outside
☐ Feel moderately or extremely stressed	☐ Make time for friends
☐ Stay home, don't engage with people	☐ Volunteer or socialize
☐ Watch more than 2 hours of TV	☐ Learn new skills or do something that challenges my brain
☐ Don't do any activity I enjoy (hobby)	☐ Pursue a hobby or do something that feels like play
☐ Think negatively about getting old	☐ Feel positive about getting older
☐ Avoid going to the doctor	☐ Make and keep appointments for checkups and screenings
☐ Avoid going to the dentist	☐ Get teeth cleaned twice a year
☐ Feel pessimistic about the future	☐ Feel excited about the future

Age Accelerants	Age Decelerants
☐ Feel adrift, wondering what my purpose is	☐ Feel connected to a sense of purpose
☐ Worry about not saving/investing enough for 3+ decades of retirement	☐ Live within my means now and invest so I'll have more financial resources later

Age accelerant total: Age decelerant total:

Step two: Take a look at your totals. If you have more accelerants than decelerants, you're by no means alone—remember, only 53 percent of women tend to actually do the things they know they need to do to age agelessly. Ideally, you'd only have one or at most two check marks in the age accelerant column and have only one or two items in the age decelerant column that *aren't* checked. If you're nowhere near those results—that's what this book can help you with. It's time to get going.

Looking at your answers, what's one aging accelerant you can minimize or stop doing altogether? And what's a decelerant you can lean in to or start doing? Choose something you can do fairly easily, to give yourself a quick win. That progress will energize you to keep making other changes as you move through this book.

THE GOAL OF AGELESS
AGING: SQUARING THE CURVE

On a long-life journey, two essential goals are to prevent or delay age-related decline and maintain health and vitality as long as possible. It's what scientists call squaring the curve, so that even if your lifespan isn't longer (although it likely will be for most of us), your years of health and vitality are—years in which you can enjoy your longevity bonus.

But, to be frank, squaring the curve won't happen just because you read a book about it. It will take effort on your part.

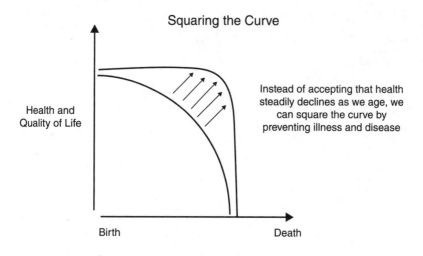

Squaring the Curve

Health and Quality of Life

Instead of accepting that health steadily declines as we age, we can square the curve by preventing illness and disease

Birth

Death

Throughout this book, I'll be your guide, describing what aging agelessly can be, what it can look and feel like, and how it can be achieved. I'll explain the many decisions you can make to ensure not just a longer life, but a healthier and happier one as well. A crucial first step on this journey is to raise your awareness—and your appreciation—of the good things about getting older. (Yes, they exist!) Nipping any negative ideas you have about aging and getting excited about the journey ahead will help you square your curve, and it's what we're diving into next.

2

EMBRACING THE UPSIDES OF LONG LIFE

More than twenty years ago, I had the great honor of spending time with Betty Friedan, bestselling author of *The Feminine Mystique*. Together with my husband, Ken, we shared a meal at a Mexican restaurant in San Francisco, where we ate chiles rellenos and tacos and drank margaritas late into the night. At the time Betty was seventy-two and tough as nails, with lots of wisdom, power, and provocative opinions.

Once the margaritas began to do their work, I asked Betty what had motivated her to write *The Feminine Mystique* in 1963. Her answer has always stuck with me. She said she wanted women to realize that they shouldn't be measured by the metric of men. In other words, women needed their own definition of success. We all clinked our margarita glasses to that!

I then asked her the same question about her new book, *The Fountain of Age*. Her answer was similar. She wanted people to realize that as we get older, if we continue to measure ourselves by the metrics of youth, we'll always be playing a losing game.

Betty was right. It makes no sense for women to measure themselves by men, and it makes no sense for women who are fifty, sixty, seventy, or eighty to be measured or measure themselves against their (often-idealized) twenty-year-old self or any other younger woman. We need to liberate ourselves from the idea that youth is the pinnacle of life.

I want to breathe into this idea to make sure you've heard me: youth—or even age—does not need to define who you are or how you feel as your life unfolds. Yes, health, vitality, and even youthfulness are goals. We do want to prevent, delay, or minimize physical and mental decline—physical or biological aging—as much as possible. That's an essential element of ageless aging. But longevity is about far more than just slowing or halting physical and mental downturns. That's still a losing game, just a slower one.

To really change your personal experience of aging, you also need to focus on what you've gained as you've lived. As I'll cover in this chapter, those are your lessons learned, your values, your perspective, and the emotional intelligence you've accumulated, to name just a few. These are metrics that anyone who wants to age more agelessly can feel proud of—and model. The good news is that, rather than being just a downward slide, this new longevity can be an ascent. In many ways, life can and does get better.

Jane Fonda, in her eighties, thinks the way our entire society views the lifelong aging process is based on an outdated paradigm of decline and decrepitude. She says, "We're still living with the old paradigm that age is a pathology. But a more appropriate metaphor for aging is a staircase—the upward ascension of the human spirit, bringing us into wisdom, wholeness, and authenticity." That's a far better way to envision our present and future.

LIFE GETS BETTER AND BETTER

Typically, it's physical changes that we tend to focus on, and sometimes obsess over, as we live longer. Whether it's noticing that you can no longer read the menu in a dimly lit restaurant, wondering why it suddenly feels ten degrees warmer in the room and no one else seems to notice (hello, hot flash!), or noticing the small lines around your eyes, it's easy to focus on the physical changes of aging. (I'll admit, I'm not the skier I used to be.) But doing so is only one side of the equation.

Nadia Tuma-Weldon, whom you met in the previous chapter, headed up a research program for McCann Worldgroup called "The Truth About Aging" to discover more about people's attitudes toward getting older. Nadia told me, "One of the main findings is that as we move through life, life gets better and better and better, particularly for women."

Let's unravel a few of the threads of why it gets better for so many women. For one thing, as we live longer, our mental health and emotional intelligence often improve. So do our confidence, our resilience, our sense of perspective and outlook on life, and even our positivity.

When we obsess less over the decline of our body, we can begin to appreciate more the growing power and resilience of our mind. And that is truly is something to celebrate.

I didn't just dream this up. During the early months of COVID, in partnership with Edward Jones and the Harris Poll, at Age Wave we began conducting multiple in-depth surveys involving more than ten thousand respondents across five generations in the United States and Canada. We were quite surprised to see that it was not younger people but older ones who displayed the most emotional and mental resilience and even well-being throughout the tumultuous times of 2020 and 2021.[1]

Think about it. It's the more mature and seasoned among us who have lived through life's ups and downs and learned that most things have a way of sorting themselves out. Situations may turn around. New possibilities may open even during times of unprecedented challenge. After all, you don't get to age fifty, sixty, seventy, and beyond without experiencing some heavy stuff—personal, professional, and in the world at large. Resilience can be the result of coping with life's trials. It truly is one of the great upsides of a long life.

Dr. Judith Rodin, psychologist, former president of the University of Pennsylvania and then the Rockefeller Foundation, and author of *The Resilience Dividend*, believes that resilience is a learned skill that can be taught, developed, and practiced. It's a muscle that, as we live longer lives, we are often forced to flex.

For instance, Elyse Pellman, president of Age Wave, and one of my very closest friends, is sixty-nine years old. She has lived with type 1 diabetes since she was in her late twenties. Type 1 diabetes is a chronic autoimmune condition that develops when your pancreas stops producing insulin or can't produce enough insulin. (Type 2 diabetes is the kind we hear about more often because it's more common and is closely associated with diet and lifestyle.) Elyse is what's called a brittle diabetic, meaning her symptoms are very difficult to manage, with unexplained variations in blood sugar. She continually faces a variety of potentially serious long-term complications, including shorter lifespan, loss of vision, and an increased risk of developing heart disease, stroke, and eye and kidney disease. In order to manage the disease, Elyse exercises every single day, no matter what. She eats incredibly healthy and wears an insulin pump and glucose monitor. But she still has trouble controlling her insulin and blood sugar within normal ranges. It's a 24/7 job. However, without exaggeration, Elyse is the most positive person I know and enjoys a normal life. Whatever is going on, she finds a way to position it in her mind as positive, or at least something she can find a solution for in order to manage it.

I asked Elyse how she does it, and here's what she told me: "As I've lived longer and coped with a serious chronic disease, I've learned to not sweat the small stuff, and to take control of the big stuff." For instance, as a result of being a type 1 diabetic for more than thirty years, she developed diabetic retinopathy in her right eye. The fear was that she would lose her sight in that eye. She visited a specialist and began taking monthly injections in the eye to forestall further damage and hopefully minimize the problem. While Elyse was extremely scared of getting that first injection directly into her eye, she did everything possible to relax. As it turned out, the worry was worse than the shot.

THE U-CURVE OF HAPPINESS

There is more good news that comes when we step out of our ageist bubbles and evaluate some of the advantages of our longer lives. The truth is, overall, as shown in study after study, once we hit our fifties and beyond, most of us report feeling happier and having greater life satisfaction than those who are younger. In fact, the sweet spot for happiness has been identified as being from about age fifty to seventy-five. Based on large-scale research conducted on Americans and Europeans, there's what's called a "U-curve of happiness" that starts out high in our youth, dips between the ages of twenty-five and fifty, then goes up again and soars in our fifties and beyond, until it turns down a bit in our eighties.[2]

Laura Carstensen, founder and director of Stanford's Longevity Center and author of *A Long Bright Future*, told me, "Younger and older people are happier and have greater life satisfaction than people in the middle. And women have more highs and lows than men. It may seem obvious, but as we women live longer without child-raising responsibilities, we're freer to do a lot of things we've always dreamed of doing with fewer restrictions on our time and our effort."

Our research at Age Wave confirms that, in general, happiness and a sense of freedom start rising appreciably around age fifty-five while anxiety plummets. This is likely influenced by, as Dr. Carstensen pointed out, predictable life-stage events such as a downshift in parenting as children grow into adults and often leave the nest.

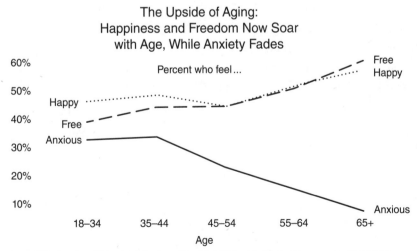

The Upside of Aging:
Happiness and Freedom Now Soar
with Age, While Anxiety Fades

Source: "The New Age of Aging: A Landmark Age Wave Study," U.S. adults 18+, top 3 box on scale of 1–10, 2023

A LIFT IN SELF-CONFIDENCE IN THE FREEDOM ZONE

It's not just happiness and life satisfaction that rise for many, but also self-confidence. Research published in the *Harvard Business Review* found that women's self-confidence may start lower than men's, but it steadily improves throughout the decades, so as we head into our sixties and beyond, we have more self-confidence than men and more than we ever had before.[3]

That means that we women are experiencing higher-than-ever levels of self-confidence as we enter what my Age Wave team has identified and labeled the *freedom zone*.

In our focus groups, we have asked what words come to mind when you think about life after fifty, sixty, or seventy, and what we heard more often than not was the word *freedom*. Both freedom *from* the stress and time requirements of raising kids, commuting, and devoting so many hours to work, and freedom *to* reinvent yourself, follow your dreams, improve your health, and spend more time with family and friends. Psychologist Jim Bramson described it this way: "There's this whole new sense of freedom, similar to that sense you have in your twenties when life is in front of you, filled with potentially unlimited opportunities, and you aren't locked into decisions. You don't have to follow a script. It's empowering, especially for women."

There are now all around us multiplying examples of women in the second half of life making the most of their freedom zone, whether it's Nancy Pelosi wielding the gavel as Speaker of the House when she was in her eighties, Viola Davis leading a tribe of female warriors in *The Woman King* at fifty-seven, or actor/model Andie MacDowell, at sixty-four, strutting her stuff on the runways in Paris during Fashion Week with her wild mane of gray curls. MacDowell described the feeling of walking the Paris runways like this: "I enjoy being glamorous now more than I ever have." She also said that her managers had advised her against going gray (something she did while in the lockdown phase of the COVID pandemic). She told them, "I think you're wrong, and I'm going to be more powerful if I embrace where I am right now."[4]

It turns out she was right. The crowds loved it and loved her. That's self-confidence in action!

Indeed, when I reached out to Emmy, Grammy, Oscar, and Tony winner Rita Moreno to be interviewed for this chapter, she replied that she was honored to be asked but that she had to be diligent with her time. She was ninety years old then, and surprised and delighted to be in such demand. "I am up to my chin in work, Zoom interviews, shooting films, and various projects that want my participation," she told me. "Who woulda thunk there would be so much interest in me at this late stage of my life?" she wrote.

New Beginnings for Women over Fifty

- Toni Morrison wrote her first novel, *The Bluest Eye*, when she was forty. She won a Pulitzer at fifty-six, and a Nobel Prize in Literature at sixty-two.

- Kris Jenner pitched her first TV show, *Keeping Up with the Kardashians*, when she was fifty-two.

- Julia Child was fifty when her first cookbook, *Mastering the Art of French Cooking*, was published.

- Betty White didn't achieve icon status until she was cast on *The Mary Tyler Moore Show* at age fifty, and her popularity soared until her final days at ninety-nine.

- Laura Ingalls Wilder published her first book, *Little House in the Big Woods*, at age sixty-four.

- Maxine Waters was first elected as a congresswoman for California at age fifty-two.

- Arianna Huffington started *The Huffington Post* when she was fifty-five and Thrive Media at sixty-six.

- Dr. Ruth Westheimer was fifty-two when she got her first radio show, *Sexually Speaking*.

> - Kathryn Bigelow became the first woman to win an Oscar for Best Director for her film *The Hurt Locker* at fifty-seven.
> - Vera Wang started designing clothes at age forty.
> - Deb Haaland became the first Native American to serve as a cabinet secretary at age sixty.

Plenty of women who aren't in the spotlight are just as inspirational. After Mary Rawles, a schoolteacher living in Novato, California, retired when she was in her sixties, she recognized that she had some worrisome health issues that she needed to educate herself about and act on. She went on a serious health kick, losing more than twenty pounds, and designed a fitness program for herself that improved not only her physical health, but also her emotional well-being. At age seventy-three, right in the middle of the pandemic, she took a leap of faith to start her own business to take what she had learned and offer it to other women: online workout classes and nutritional support. Mary said she'd always wanted to start her own business, but she didn't have the confidence to go for it until she was in her seventies.

Another example is Denise Kaufman. Back in 1967, during the Summer of Love, Denise, together with four other women, formed one of the first all-female rock bands, called Ace of Cups. They opened for Jimi Hendrix the week after his groundbreaking performance at the Monterey Pop Festival. Hendrix went back to London raving about Ace of Cups to anyone who would listen. As a result, bands like Jefferson Airplane and the Grateful Dead hired them as their opening act and helped to make them a local sensation in the San Francisco psychedelic music scene. However, they were never able to get a record deal or a national tour. According to Denise, "We played for the sake of music, not for the sake of stardom. Plus we couldn't be easily pigeonholed. We didn't wear matching outfits like other girl bands. We were told that we were too raw, yet we were playing the same kind of music as the guy bands. It was very frustrating." Unfortunately, they eventually gave up their dream of getting a record deal or gaining a national following.

Five decades later, that all changed. A producer came across some of their rehearsal tapes as well as live performances from back in the day and loved their sound. He wanted to release their music. Four of the five original band members regrouped and reemerged as rock stars. In fact, they actually got their first record deal, got lots of positive press, and even performed live on the *Today* show . . . in their seventies. Ace of Cups still lives on, and the group is planning their next album release. They are finally living their dream to be female rock stars in their eighth decade of life.

A DIFFERENT KIND OF AFFLUENCE: LONGEVITY'S TIME AFFLUENCE

Denise Kaufman's dreams wouldn't have come true if her life had been shorter. They also would have been a lot more challenging to realize while she was still in the middle of raising her daughter and taking on the responsibilities of earning a living. It was only later in life that she had the bandwidth to pivot and pursue her lifelong dream. This points to another upside of long life, known as *time affluence*: when we hit our sixth decade of life and beyond, we often have more free time. For an increasing number of older women, this is a time to try new things, pursue interests we've always wanted to pursue but didn't have the time for, or reinvent ourselves in some new ways. We can be beginners again.

Take Quin Bommelje, who was involved with tennis for more than thirty years, first as a player, then as a teacher, and finally as a coach for her son's high school team. But when she noticed a cut on her lip and a spot on her scalp that wouldn't heal, she went to the dermatologist, who told her to stay completely out of the sun because these were precancerous lesions. Quin quit tennis immediately, which put her into a serious funk.

At this point Quin was sixty years old and now had a lot of time on her hands. She wasn't sure what to do with all this time affluence. Not long after, one of her son's friends was getting married. His parents told

Quin that they were going to take dance lessons so they could enjoy the wedding even more. Quin had never danced a step in her life but thought it might be fun to try. So she went home and convinced her husband to take dance lessons with her: "That way we could have more fun at the wedding, move around instead of sitting around watching everyone else dance." They signed up for ten lessons at Arthur Murray Dance School.

At first Quin couldn't even keep a beat, and her husband and their instructor cringed as they watched her dance. But she really wanted to learn, so she stuck with it. And she was persistent, even after her husband lost interest and quit.

Fast-forward a decade, and at age seventy-one, Quin is still dancing, but now as a competitive ballroom dancer. Together with her thirty-five-year-old partner, Misha Vlasov, she appeared in 2018 on NBC's *America's Got Talent*, choking up the judges with her amazing performance. Martina McBride told her and the audience, "You say you want to inspire people of a certain age, but you have inspired everybody of all ages."

METABOLIZING YOUR EXPERIENCE TO BUILD YOUR WISDOM

Of course, it's possible to be facing big stress and life challenges at any age, and they can take a toll on your mental health and overall well-being. It's precisely these tough experiences, though, that can sometimes build our emotional resilience and even create wisdom over time. Chip Conley, founder and former CEO of Joie de Vivre Hospitality, senior advisor to the founders of Airbnb, board member of Burning Man and Esalen Institute, and more recently creator of Modern Elder Academy—which is devoted to helping people at midlife and beyond discover a renewed sense of purpose and "reframe your midlife from a crisis to a calling"—offered me a definition of wisdom that I found insightful: "Wisdom is metabolized experience that leads to distilled compassion."

Let's break this down. First, wisdom is different from knowledge. The internet adds 2.5 quintillion bytes of knowledge every day; while some of the things posted online are decidedly frivolous in nature, and misinformation—anti-knowledge—is also uploaded every day, facts and figures are at our fingertips like never before.

Wisdom, on the other hand, is something we develop within ourselves. It's the ability to discern patterns, and that pattern recognition comes from experience—if you've experienced something before, you know more about how to deal with it. But just because you've experienced something doesn't mean that you've learned from it or metabolized it. I'm sure you've observed someone in your life—maybe it's you—repeating the same missteps over and over.

When you've processed an experience, can review it objectively, and are no longer triggered into a big emotional reaction by it, you have metabolized it. As you mature, you gain insight you can then use to reduce suffering for yourself and others. That's distilled compassion. This compassion could be channeled toward yourself— creating emotional stability, reinventing yourself, or reworking a no-longer-tenable situation—or toward helping others solve challenges in their lives.

New generations of older women are increasingly seeking out ways to metabolize their experiences and shape their wisdom. For example, 62 percent of the people who enroll at Conley's Modern Elder Academy—workshops and online programs explicitly designed to help people at midlife and beyond to cultivate and harvest their wisdom and reinvent themselves—are women. Yet, Conley says that he's noticed that women are less inclined than men to call themselves wise. Ironically, this tendency speaks to women's age-related maturity. "It shows how wise women are, because, generally, humility is an important part of wisdom," he told me.

Of course, there's no shame in owning your wisdom. Another thing Rita Moreno told me is, "The best part of aging for me is how wise I've become. And smart!" When I asked what she attributed that to, she replied, "I suppose you could say that I've experienced a lot, and

I've learned to listen very well." And listening is something that will help you keep learning and building your wisdom, too.

GENERATIVITY AND THE RISE OF THE MENTERN

Having opportunities to share your wisdom is another terrific benefit of getting older. "Being able to repurpose your wisdom for your own benefit is great, but it's even better when you can repurpose it for the benefit of other people," Conley told me. "You take the seed of what you've learned and plant it in different soil," which is exactly what Conley did when he signed on as a mentor to the founders of Airbnb and transferred the wisdom he had accumulated as the founder of Joie de Vivre Hospitality to help skyrocket Airbnb to success.

What surprised Conley about being the oldest person in the office at Airbnb is how much he had to learn from the younger professionals he was mentoring. "I was learning as much from them as they were from me," he told me, so he labeled what he was doing "menterning"—a combination of mentoring and interning.

We needn't restrict building a give-and-take relationship with people of other age brackets to the workplace. Ashton Applewhite calls intergenerational friendships "an anti-ageism life hack"—which is why I've included it in the hack section at the end of this chapter. "If more older women had younger friends as well as friends even older than they are, we would all be reminded of both the joys and challenges of every stage of life," she points out.

I've taken Ashton's advice to heart. Over the last several years, I've gone out of my way to create relationships with women of different ages. It began by befriending some of my daughter Casey's friends. We traveled with a group of her thirtysomething friends before COVID and now get together with them for dinner or just a Zoom meet-up on a regular basis. I have also befriended a friend of my son Zak's, fortysomething Dana Griffin, marketer extraordinaire and founder/ CEO of Eldera (Elder.ai), an online platform that connects kids from around the globe with vetted older adult mentors. Dana, who was raised in Transylvania (now a part of Romania), is bold, playful, and smart as a whip. She's also deeply committed to helping older adults share their wisdom with the world. We had a lot of common interests in terms of our work and started spending time together without any of Zak's involvement. I love the fact that we each bring fresh perspectives to discussions yet enjoy a lot of the same work and life activities.

My friendships with these younger women have introduced me to new lingo, ideas, and music that I might never have experienced without having them in my life. It has helped me feel both more culturally engaged and far more alive.

PLUSSING THE NEGATIVES

A way to improve the narrative of a tough situation and turn it into a positive learning experience and maybe even a nugget of wisdom is to look for opportunities to do what is called "plussing." I first heard this term over two decades ago from Dave Zaboski, a friend and my co-author of the children's book *Gideon's Dream: A Tale of New Beginnings*. Dave worked as a senior animator on *The Lion King* and *Beauty and the Beast* at Disney, where he was taught that there are no bad ideas. In workshop sessions at Disney, his groups would work through creative ideas by taking what was presented (even if you didn't like the idea to begin with), finding the positive in it, and improving it in some way. It's what they called "plussing."

Let's borrow this notion of plussing and relate it to our own efforts at self-improvement. For example, say you are having trouble sleeping—something that could easily take a chunk out of your happiness. But you do your research (including reading Chapter 6 of this book, where we'll cover sleep in depth) and decide to turn this problem into a positive. You might begin by discussing a magnesium supplement—which is commonly recommended to promote sleep as it is a relaxant—with your doctor, to make sure there are no contraindications for you (such as IBS or kidney disease). If she agrees it's a good fit, the magnesium may also help remedy constipation (because it is a relaxant that also helps to relax the muscles of the digestive tract). Since magnesium is known as a relaxant for the nervous system as well, you might notice you feel a little calmer, too. In addition, you could be addressing a mineral deficiency you didn't even know you had (at least 50 percent of all Americans are deficient in magnesium) and boosting your overall health, as magnesium deficiency is linked to an increased risk for cardiovascular disease, diabetes, and osteoporosis.[5] *That* is a definite plus.

THE POSITIVITY EFFECT

An important piece of the resilience that we tend to accrue as we live longer is what researchers refer to as the *positivity effect*—the tendency to pay more attention to positive news and information. This is the exact opposite of what's known as the negativity bias—the tendency to focus on and remember more acutely negative news and experiences, and something that tends to rule our attention in our twenties, thirties, and forties.

Dr. Laura Carstensen explained the positivity effect to me like this: "As we see time running out in our fifties, our sixties, our seventies, it becomes increasingly clear to us that we're not going to be here forever, and so we might say, 'I want to make the most of it. I don't want to get tied up in these trivial matters that drive people crazy when they're young.' Instead, older adults are more focused in the present. So there is something about aging that I think is really a gift."

This present-moment awareness helps us access a range of positive emotions, such as gratitude, appreciation, and resilience. These emotional states then help us recalibrate our priorities so that we spend time on what we are thankful for and appreciate the *now*—and not put off things until some point in the future. Dr. Carstensen added, "Ideally, older people can also think about the long-term future, and apply their wisdom, concerns, and investments to that long-term future. At the same time, we have less desire to devote energy to things that *don't* matter—primarily, what other people think about us."

BEING MORE, WHILE CARING
LESS WHAT OTHER PEOPLE THINK

One of the biggest fears of aging, especially for women, is invisibility. And yes, if you have been accustomed to turning heads when you walk into a room, it can feel like a loss to no longer have the attention and energy of desirability directed your way. But there is also power and a sense of freedom in it. Ashton Applewhite described it to me this way: "I can do what I want without worrying about what the hot straight guy at the bar might think of me. He's never going to pay attention to me, so I'm not going to waste a nanosecond trying to get his attention." Maybe that's the subtle art of not giving a shit, but as we mature, we know we have far better places to put our energy than just obsessing about how we look to others.

Authenticity and self-awareness are also gifts that often come with living a long life. Many women report that they now feel more comfortable in their own skin, even if it has a few more wrinkles. Seventy-nine-year-old actor Helen Mirren put it this way: "When you're young and beautiful, you're paranoid and miserable. I think one of the great advantages of getting older is that you let go of these kinds of things."

CHANGING THE CULTURAL NARRATIVE:
A GIFT TO THE NEXT GENERATIONS

Recognizing and appreciating the many upsides of aging is an essential ingredient to approaching longevity with a more positive mindset, which we know can influence our healthspan and our lifespan. And when we change our own inner narrative to place higher value on these upsides, it will also help change the cultural narrative regarding what is possible for women as they live longer. This is a gift to ourselves and also a gift to future generations of women.

I believe those of us in our fifties, sixties, seventies, and beyond need to share the news that getting older doesn't have to be scary. Describing her research at Truth Central, Nadia Tuma-Weldon said, "The data in our studies have shown that aging is a bigger problem for the young, because it seems so scary. It seems like the great unknown." She also told me that "young people really love when older women are featured in advertising and marketing because it makes them feel really positive about their own aging. And not just from a physical perspective." She gave me this example: "I was scrolling through Instagram, and I saw a post about Kimiko Nishimoto, a ninety-four-year-old Japanese woman. She's a photographer, and there was a carousel of her incredible photographs. The caption read, '94-year-old started her photography career at age 72.' And there were thousands and thousands of likes, thousands of comments. People love these stories that just aren't told enough about women who live long lives and have a great story to tell." She went on to say, "What I've learned, and what young people need to hear, is it's not just about the length of life, but the depth of life!"

As we age more agelessly, we can collectively embrace the gifts of aging and the idea that living longer can be beautiful. In the process, we can become role models to younger generations for what their lives can be as they hit their fifties, sixties, seventies, eighties, nineties, and beyond. Joan Ditzion, a member of the Boston Women's Health Book Collective and co-author of the seminal book on women's health *Our Bodies, Ourselves*, told me one of the most important things we can do to feel more positive about getting older and to inspire younger women to feel the same is to "honor the diversity of experiences, change the narrative of what it means to age, and make it normative." In other words, to talk about our experiences and share our points of view, just like the consciousness-raising talks that women in the 1970s embraced as part of feminism's second wave. After all, we are the first generation in history to live such long lives en masse—and to live them with health, power, and purpose. Let's pass on the knowledge and wisdom we've gained to pave the way for those who will come after us, and share everything we learn about to have both longer lives and deeper lives.

EMBRACING THE UPSIDE OF
LONG LIFE: WHERE TO BEGIN

If you do one thing: Push back against ageist assumptions

One of the things that drives me up a wall is when people learn how old I am and tell me, "Wow, you look *so good* for your age!" I know they mean well, but it reveals their own internalized ageism that tries to tell them that older people are not supposed to be attractive. When I spoke to Ashton Applewhite, she shared a comeback line I love: "Thanks! You look great for your age, too!" We have to—playfully—call out each other's ageist assumptions; it's the only way we'll start to challenge them and rewrite the script.

If you're a total beginner: Make friends
with someone older *and* someone younger

A great way to share your upsides of aging with others—and to help dissolve the invisible, and ageist, dividers between the generations—is to form friendships with people of all ages. Applewhite told me, "If more younger women had older friends, they would realize how age is a source of power, self-knowledge, and confidence. They would be less afraid of getting older, and they would realize how much of our youth we squander on worrying about this shit."

This will require some effort, as it goes against the tide. Research shows that age segregation is as pervasive as racial segregation. And ageism is at play here—some young people dismiss older people, while older people may judge younger adults. Older adults can also definitely judge themselves, believing that younger people don't want to talk to them simply because of their age. Put that positivity effect and rising self-confidence to use: stop telling yourself that someone is too old or too young to become friends with, and open yourself up to intergenerational friendships.

— ◆ —

If you're already embracing the upside of aging and are ready
to take it to the next level: Become a mentern

Finding ways to share your accumulated knowledge helps you give back
and find your own sense of purpose. You'll also probably develop some
intergenerational relationships while you're at it, while also keeping
yourself exposed to new ideas. If being a mentor holds appeal for you,
there are numerous organizations that help you plug in and give back
in a meaningful way to people who are significantly younger than you.
They include Marc Freedman's CoGenerate, which seeks to bridge the
age divide and bring multiple generations together to solve the world's
problems (cogenerate.org); Eldera, which matches older adults with
children to mentor (eldera.ai); the Experience Corps, which trains volunteers who are fifty and over to tutor kids in public elementary schools
(aarp.com/experience-corps); Big and Mini, which matches older adults
with younger adults to bridge the generational divide (bigandmini.org);
Hey Auntie, which connects older women of color with their younger
counterparts (heyauntie.io); and SCORE, a network of volunteer business mentors who help fledgling entrepreneurs (score.org). Or join a
corporate, nonprofit, or community board. If you're working for or
running a company, you can ask HR about setting up a program to
pair mentors and mentees—perhaps you'll learn that there is already
one that you didn't know about. And if you're no longer working, or
work for yourself, think about who's already in your network who is of
a different generation. You can invite them to coffee or a Zoom call and
say, "I want to learn more about what you're working on and where
you want to go from here." It's almost like dating.

AGELESS AGING HACKS
TO EMBRACE THE UPSIDE OF AGING

Raise your awareness of your own ageism . . . and the ageism
of those around you

We can't challenge bias unless we're aware of it, and most bias is
unconscious. To raise awareness of your own ageist thoughts, start

looking at your own use of the words *old* and *young*, and whether you talk about older adults as "them" or "us."

To take it a step further, talk to friends and family members about your collective experiences with ageism—both external and internal. When you talk to other women about your experiences, you realize, "Oh, these are not just my personal problems—these are widely shared political and social problems, and we can come together and do something about them." Not only can that inspire and empower you, but also these conversations are how we start to change cultural assumptions about getting older.

Attend—or host—a Generations Over Dinner gathering

Chip Conley's Modern Elder Academy has launched a program to foster age-spanning friendships. It's called Generations Over Dinner, and it guides individuals on how to gather a group of people of different generations. It also provides a series of thought-provoking questions for participants to answer, to help foster communication and connection. "What we hear over and over again from people who have organized these dinners is, 'Wow, that was life-changing,'" Conley told me. You can find more information and get started forming your own group—or joining one that already exists near you—at generationsoverdinner.com. Or you can host your own dinner with people of different ages that you are already connected to but perhaps haven't socialized with in a group before.

Listen to music "the kids" are listening to

It's a stereotype that each generation hates—or just doesn't understand—the music of the younger generations, and that we tend to keep listening to the same artists we discovered in our teens and twenties for the rest of our lives. An analysis of listening habits of users of the streaming platform Spotify found that after age thirty-three, we tend to stop listening to new (as in recently produced) music.[6]

Research shows that there is a link between listening to new music and open-mindedness—it helps establish new neural pathways as you become familiar with the different rhythms and chord progressions.[7] "New music listening activates areas of the brain from root to tip, from the early auditory processing centers to the outer reaches of our cortex," says Victoria Williamson, music psychology professor and author of *You Are the Music*. Because listening to new music styles is so stimulating to the brain, and pop music is such a great shared cultural reference, make it a point to listen to music that is currently popular. It's a great way to expand your horizons and connect to younger people.

Ask your kids or grandkids for recommendations, tune your car radio to the local pop station, or look for "new and noteworthy" playlists on your streaming platform. And don't be quick to reject it. Try to learn what it means, why it's popular, and with whom.

Prepare for takeoff

Actively imagine the rise in your happiness, self-confidence, and life satisfaction that will follow when you develop a more positive viewpoint on your own ageless aging. Allow yourself to be optimistic about the future and honest about your hopes and dreams, and let these ideas inspire you and help you see new possibilities. Remember that the positivity effect builds resilience, and metabolized experiences fuel you in making a plan for exactly how you will maximize your longevity bonus.

3

◆

CHARTING YOUR PATH

In a perfect world, you'd have a GPS system to guide you through countless choices, detours, and possible bumps in the road on your ageless aging journey. Plug in the destination, a route is optimized for you, and Siri tells you when to turn left at the drugstore, right at the gym, and so on. Unfortunately, it doesn't work like that (yet).

What you can do today is design your own unique path, complete with knowing what pitfalls to avoid, tips and techniques to take advantage of, hacks to try out, and fun to have along the way. In other words, you need a plan—and you've come to the right place. Keep in mind that the plan will evolve and change as you, and your life, evolves and changes. In this chapter, you'll learn the 5 steps to charting your course successfully.

They are:

1. Identify your intention/action gap(s).
2. Create your vision.
3. Identify your entry point.
4. Make a plan.
5. Course-correct.

Although there are clearly defined steps, for now, the path to ageless aging is more recipe than map. Start with the basics, fold in more ingredients to enhance the recipe, and watch how everything interacts to create an amazing result: a healthy, agelessly aging you.

THE POWER OF SMALL STEPS

I think of the recipe for ageless aging as a kind of stone soup, an image from a European folk tale that tells the story of hungry travelers coming to a village with nothing but an empty pot. Those travelers put a stone in the pot, filled it with water, and set it over a fire. As residents came by to ask what was in the pot, they said it was a stone soup that would be made even tastier if everyone could share a little garnish. Each villager shared a little bit of food to add to the pot, resulting in a delicious soup that fed everyone (after removing the stone, of course). This parable shows not only the benefits of sharing, but also that little contributions add up to something nourishing, and that a wide variety of ingredients can work together synergistically, interacting with each other, enhancing each other, and creating a whole that is greater than the sum of its parts.

This isn't just the stuff of fairy tales—by customizing your own recipe and then committing yourself to implement those changes, you can influence both your healthspan and lifespan more dramatically than any one single ingredient could do on its own. Any particular step you take or ingredient you add may not seem like much, but they can come together to create something great.

When I spoke with Dr. Stephen Kopecky, the Mayo Clinic cardiologist I first introduced in Chapter 1, he said that most people don't understand the power of small steps. "Every single patient I talk to is looking for one of two things—they either want the single drug, supplement, exercise, or superfood that would transform their health, or they come in and say, 'Doc, I want to change everything. I'm going to do everything differently.'" The problem with both of these common approaches is that neither one of them works. "It's never just one thing," Kopecky told me. "It has to be a series of very small changes in multiple areas over time." But I believe you need to start with just one step at a time.

That "over time" piece is important, too, especially for women. Depending on how old you are now, you still have multiple decades in front of you—maybe four, five, or even six decades. Think about how the benefits of any little changes you make now can compound over time. Steady wins the race.

To reap those long-term benefits, and to move from powerless to powerful, a plan is needed. Let's start creating your plan with this first step.

STEP 1: IDENTIFY YOUR INTENTION/ACTION GAPS

Remember the intention/action gap I introduced in Chapter 1? We often know what to do—too many of us just don't take the steps to do it. That's why I included the Self-Assessment in Chapter 1, so that you can start to tease out both what you're already doing well—which is important, as you want to celebrate your wins—but also get very clear on the health-promoting things you're *not* doing, as well as the potentially harmful things that you *are* doing.

When I interviewed Dr. Suzanne Steinbaum, a New York City cardiologist and author of *Dr. Suzanne Steinbaum's Heart Book: Every Woman's Guide to a Heart-Healthy Life*, she said the first step she always tells her patients who want to get healthier is to conduct an audit of their current habits. It's essential not only for knowing what needs changing, but also for discovering your motivation to change.

"If you don't look at your whole life and take a ruthless analysis of those things that are on the pro side, that really support your health, versus the con side, things that do not support your health, you don't really have an understanding of how to move forward and how to make those changes," she told me.

One of her patients, who was trying to lose weight, told her the only time she had to catch up on laundry was at night after her kids were in bed. She often snacked as she did those chores, as a way to treat herself. She was stuck in a loop of thinking, "I have to do the laundry at night, and I have to snack in order to make doing the laundry more tolerable. There's no other way."

"When she described to me what was happening," Dr. Steinbaum related, "I said, 'Let's take a look at that snacking. Write down everything you eat.'" Turns out, this woman was eating about 1,500 calories after nine o'clock on most nights. Dr. Steinbaum said to her, "Here's my prescription for you: go to bed earlier." Three months later, this patient had lost fifteen pounds, not because she radically changed her diet, but because she became aware of the habit pattern she had that wasn't working for her and began making small changes. She started doing laundry on a weekend morning, for one thing. And she did indeed get to bed earlier most nights. What made those changes possible was changing the story she told herself. Instead of thinking, "If I don't stay up all night and do the laundry and snack, my family is not going to be taken care of," she began telling herself a truer story, which was, "I have to just go to bed and take care of myself and figure out a better time to do laundry."

It's that self-honesty that brings more self-awareness. It's the first step to bridging your own intention/action gap. Raising your awareness is not something you do once, when you're doing an initial audit of your current habits and actions, but something you continue to practice. If I'm about to pick up a piece of cake with a big thick layer of frosting on it, I try to be aware of what I'm doing, telling myself that the cake is a treat, and, if I choose to indulge, savoring every bite. I'm also going to be really aware of how I feel the next day, so that I can assess whether that treat was really worth it. It usually isn't.

Another hugely important piece of awareness to raise is about your own future. Because although all the things you can do to take care of yourself will definitely help you feel better and be happier *now*, they will also multiply or compound over time and set you up for a much better reality in the future. I think of it as *taking control of your future self*.

A top reason why the intention/action gap is so big, especially for women in their forties and fifties, is often because they're busy taking care of everyone else and putting themselves last on their to-do lists. They think, "I'll pay more attention to this after the kids leave home, or when I retire." That kind of thinking sacrifices your future self.

It's time to start telling yourself a different, truer story. Here's one, from Cassie Holmes, author of *Happier Hour* and a UCLA professor of marketing and behavior decision-making: "The pursuit of one's own personal happiness and satisfaction is not frivolous or selfish, because when we take care of ourselves, it allows us to show up better for other people and whatever we do in our lives." Beyond that, "when you invest time in things that fill you up, you increase your sense of self-efficacy and your experience of positive emotions that then make you feel like you have more time."

When you identify one or two or more ingredients that you could add to your stone soup, then close your intention/action gap by actually doing them, you nurture your present self and your future self. You'll feel better now, and when you get to your sixty-fifth, seventieth, or eighty-fifth birthday, you also get to realize, "Wow, I'm so thankful that I did those things for myself that set me up so well." And along the way, you'll feel that you have more time and more agency over how you spend that time.

For example, if you start investing a little more money after reading Chapter 11 of this book (which I sincerely hope you will), by the time you get to sixty-five, seventy, or eighty-five, you'll be in a much better position to consider taking time off from work and less likely to be forced to keep working forty hours a week to have enough money to live. Whatever steps you choose to take may require some trade-offs; you may have to forgo some fancy dinners or choose a more affordable vacation so you can invest more. But you can still enjoy yourself on the journey, and investing more can alleviate your anxiety about your future, which can help you feel better now *and* later. You don't need to deprive yourself; just make some potential trade-offs.

It comes down to raising your awareness as a first step. Cassie Holmes suggests a simple yet effective way of doing this that can be applied to almost any kind of change: "If you want to lose weight, keep a food diary. If you want to get out of debt, record your spending. Likewise, if you want to invest your time better, keep track of how you're currently spending it." This helps you see clearly the size and scope of what you want to change.

STEP 2: CREATE YOUR VISION,
FIND YOUR BLISS POINT

In his bestselling book *The 4-Hour Workweek*, author Tim Ferriss famously said, "People would rather be unhappy than uncertain." Choosing to change means that things *can* change, and while that is likely to be an improvement, the fact that it would be *new* means it would also be uncertain. One kink in our wiring is that our brains register uncertainty the same way they register mistakes. Uncertainty— and change—makes us uncomfortable. Embracing change can feel scary, but it is also an opportunity to be happier, healthier, and more comfortable in your own skin.

Another thing that can make change feel more doable is getting crystal clear on what you're trying to create: your intention or goal. DeEtte Sauer, the master swimmer you met in Chapter 1, describes her ultimate goal as a "bliss point." That's a term used in the food industry to describe the perfect mixture of sweet, savory, and fat that tastes so good, it creates a form of euphoria that is addictive. I find the way DeEtte defines the term to be utterly inspiring and empowering: "I believe that we have to create a bliss point for aging, and what we want that to feel and look like. That means having stability in spiritual, physical, financial, social, and emotional areas of your life. When those come together, that's a bliss point."

What I love about the bliss point is that it encourages you to do the things that both make you feel good now and will help lead you to a future where you continue to grow in that bliss.

So, what does your bliss point look and feel like? Spend time dreaming, writing, thinking, and talking about how you really want to feel. Dr. Jim Bramson told me that "journaling is really essential for making change happen at any age, because it's a very effective method for getting in touch with the changes that you want to make, based on who you are and what you value."

What are the things you've always dreamed of doing that you haven't done? What things do you value? Is it travel, spending time with family, your financial health, or something else? How do you want to feel in your body? In your mind? Write all these things down and build a mental picture of what your bliss point looks like so that you know what you're aiming for.

Once you've got the clear vision, your work is to believe in your ability to manifest it. The word *manifestation* means to create something or turn something from an idea into a reality. The idea behind it is a little woo-woo, but it is based on the notion that you attract what you are focused on. I think there's some truth to that. Whatever is top of mind for you is what you will pay more attention to and put more energy toward.

Manifesting isn't as simple as "dream it and it will happen." You still need to do some heavy lifting. I think of it as reverse engineering. Once you can envision your bliss point clearly, you can work backward and enumerate the steps it will take to get there. Then it's a question of one foot in front of the other, again and again and again. If that sounds hard, well, it can be. But you've done hard things before—and it's not about embracing change for the sake of change or doing hard things for the sake of seeing how much you can endure. "It's being intentional about how you want your later years to feel and being willing to invest in that plan," DeEtte says. "It's not like life just happens. We get to decide how we want it to happen."

STEP 3: IDENTIFY YOUR STARTING POINT

I hope that you've done your audit (or at least the assessment I included in Chapter 1, if not both) and created your vision, and are ready to get going on your ageless aging journey. What you need now are the specific ingredients to incorporate into your holistic recipe.

Keep in mind that your journey to ageless aging starts with one change. My friend Susan is a prime example: at age fifty-five, this regular exerciser decided to up her game and try a triathlon. She didn't even know how to swim, but she wanted to test her limits and see if she could learn and combine it with two things she really enjoyed, biking and running. Fast-forward ten years, and she is now a competitive, sponsored triathlete. (Along the way, she met a fellow triathlete, fell in love, and is very happily married.)

That *one* change in Susan's life led her to make other incremental changes in her fifties and sixties. We can all do some version of this. Maybe not every woman can become a professional triathlete, whether because of mobility challenges or simply because of an utter lack of interest, and that's fine. You don't need to overcomplicate things or set an audacious goal—I've heard it said that the easy way is hard enough, and that's highly applicable here. No matter who you are, how you're wired, and what resources you have available to you, you have the power to make small changes that can take you in an unexpected—and unexpectedly delightful—direction.

By adding any ingredient, from a new exercise routine to starting a meditation practice, you will be able to set things in motion to stay more ageless. Thus far in the book, you've read about four different hacks for ageless aging—at the end of Chapter 2—and there are more to come. In each chapter, I'm also outlining where to start if you're a beginner, what to do if you can only do one thing, and how to take it to the next level if you've already got some momentum going. You could choose any of those as your first step. If you want to be more strategic, several of the experts I spoke to suggested starting by changing the most harmful thing you're doing, in order to leapfrog your health forward. Dr. Jim Bramson agreed, saying, "Whatever somebody is avoiding the most is usually where to start. If you don't want to talk about money, that's where to start. If you don't want to talk about your addiction to sweets, we're going to go there." Facing the big thing head-on reduces your anxiety and increases your self-confidence to make change happen.

All that being said, one size does not fit all. For some, starting with something that seems totally manageable is another strategy that can lead to success. Melody-Rose, a blogger I follow on Medium, wrote a post about how drinking more water changed her life. Not only did it make her feel better in the morning, help her think more clearly, and increase her sense of taste, but it also motivated her to make other healthier choices. "The little alterations I ended up making throughout the months were impacted by my one healthy choice," she wrote. She felt better, which inspired her to try exercising more, which gave her the incentive to eat better. "One thing led to another, and soon my entire lifestyle transformed in ways I didn't even plan."

Everyone I spoke with also agreed that small steps are powerful. It's the concept embodied by the Japanese word *kaizen*—that small steps lead to continuous improvement. Whatever you choose to do, take one step forward, intentionally. By making one change and feeling the benefits of that change, you can boost your confidence to experiment with other changes.

Many of the experts I spoke with suggested starting with exercise, which is where I would start as well. Why? Because just walking thirty minutes a day will make you feel better in a very short amount of time. You may have more energy, feel less sluggish, lose weight, and more . . . all in a matter of weeks. On the other hand, some experts thought changes in your diet were the easiest and best way to start. For instance, cutting out all ultra-processed foods or sugar (or both) will change how you look and feel rather quickly, inspiring you to make even more changes. Again, one size does not fit all.

It's important to note that the practice of deciding your next step will continue throughout the rest of this book and long after you've reached the final page. Each chapter in this book will introduce you to more possible ingredients, from the most basic tweaks (like flossing your teeth every night) to the cutting edge (like using contrast oxygen therapy while exercising to boost your cardiovascular and brain health) to the more pervasive changes (like weeding most or all sugar out of your diet, for real this time). But you have to start somewhere.

STEP 4: MAKE A PLAN

Getting started can be scary, but it can also be energizing. When I spoke with Nancy Katz, a career coach in Orinda, California, she explained it this way: "Initially, change is exciting. We experience a lot of motivation, but that initial rush of hope and expectation often runs out. Going into day four or day five can be complicated, as that's when the initial rush may wear off."

To get through those rough patches, you need a plan. As Cassie Holmes says, "Once you have done the work to identify what is important to you, it is absolutely about putting it into the calendar so that you are committing to it and protecting time for it." Otherwise other things can and will creep in that time you could be devoting toward your current and future self. Protecting that time by blocking it out on your calendar "allows you to be more fully engaged and remove all that thinking about all those other things you could be doing," Holmes says. When you block out time in your calendar to work on that first step, you're saying, "This is important to me."

Online transformation and personal fitness coach Caroline Drury, from Winnipeg, Canada, focuses on process, not outcome, to stay on her plan and help her clients—mostly women over fifty—do the same. She schedules her workouts in her calendar as appointments, which reinforces visually for her that this is an activity that is a priority. "I never want to let myself forget that fitness and health for my longevity are priorities in my life second only to my marriage and family," she told me.

It's also crucial to manage your own expectations. No one is going to get it right all the time, and that's okay. "Perfection is the antithesis of what you're trying to make happen because it's impossible," Katz says. Rather than getting hung up on achieving a specific goal and nailing it every step of the way, you have to embrace the process and trust that your progress will be more of an upward-trending curlicue rather than a straight line. Some days you'll do things really well, and some days you just won't.

Over time, you can even automate your progress by turning your new actions into habits. After all, as motivational author and speaker Stephen Covey says, "Our habits will either make us or break us. We become what we repeatedly do."

How then, do you build a habit? "You just have to hang in there long enough to start getting into a new reality, where the things that feel hard and new now become effortless," Katz says. In other words, they become habit. For example, it takes about four weeks for sweet foods to stop tasting so good.[1] Although you do want to make long-lasting changes, you won't always have to make long-lasting efforts.

Wendy Wood, bestselling author of *Good Habits, Bad Habits* and Provost Professor of Psychology and Business at the University of Southern California (USC), describes the practice of creating a new habit this way: "Until we have laid down a habit in neural networks and memory systems, we must willfully decide to repeat a new action again and again, even when it's a struggle. At some point, it becomes second nature, and we can sit back and let autopilot drive." Different habits will take different lengths of time to create, depending on how complex they are—one study by Pippa Lally, a researcher in Wood's lab, found that it took study participants who wanted to eat something healthy daily a total of sixty-five days for that new action to feel automatic, while those who wanted to exercise every day needed about ninety-one days for it to happen without a lot of thought. On average, no matter the desired new behavior, it took participants sixty-six days to transform something novel into old hat.[2]

You don't just have to white-knuckle it until your new behavior becomes a habit. Make it easy to do the new behavior. If you want to start eating healthier snacks and ditch the chips and cookies, stop buying the chips and cookies, place a pretty bowl of fruit on the counter, and cut up some vegetables and put them front and center in your fridge next to some hummus, so it's the first thing you see when you start looking for a nosh. If you want to exercise more, don't hide your equipment away—leave it out. Seeing it every day will help compel you to start using it. There are a few other tactics that help you lay down a new habit:

- **Friction.** In addition to making your new habit easy to do, you want to make it more difficult to do the old behavior—in other words, introduce some friction that will slow your previously automated choices. Continuing with the healthy snack example, as I said earlier, the best way to introduce friction is to stop buying the processed stuff. When my son, Zak, and his wife, FeyFey, lived with us for a few months during the pandemic, he brought his snack habits with him (we didn't call him Snack Dychtwald for nothing), and my husband and I started eating the snacks because they were there. When we discussed it as a family, we agreed to stop bringing packaged snacks into the house, and boom—snack habit interrupted.

- **Rewards.** Getting a reward for performing your new behavior helps cement the behavior in your mind, because it lights up the reward pathways in your brain (thanks, dopamine). Just be careful that you don't equate "reward" with something that could negate your ageless aging efforts, like smoking a cigarette, having multiple alcoholic beverages, or spending an afternoon mindlessly scrolling on your phone or bingeing TV.

- **Stacking.** Tie your new behavior to an existing habit. The term, first introduced in 2014 in S. J. Scott's book *Habit Stacking: 127 Small Changes to Improve Your Health, Wealth, and Happiness*, is a great way to create new habits. For example, my writing collaborator, Kate Hanley, discovered that she had osteopenia and decided to start taking bone-strengthening supplements. A devoted tea lover (with a poor track record of sticking with supplements), Kate put her pills right next to her electric kettle, so that she could tie taking her supplements to her morning cup of tea, which she never misses.

Creating a habit isn't about willpower, which is a finite resource that burns a lot of brainpower and will run out long before those sixty-six days of habit building are up. It's also not about luck, motivation, or being born a naturally healthy person. It's about devoting the time, staying committed, and embracing discipline, which might sound unappealing but can actually feel liberating. According to Jocko Willink, a former Navy SEAL and fitness expert who writes about this in his 2017 bestseller, *Discipline Equals Freedom*, discipline is a key to unlocking personal growth and success. As DeEtte Sauer puts it, "Living with discipline is my real freedom." Repeating a beneficial action until it becomes second nature is what helps you get to that bliss point. "A lot of decisions are difficult in the moment," DeEtte says, "but what's coming as a result of those choices is better. Stay focused on the rewards."

What Keeps You on Track?

Here are five ways to make it easier—and possibly even fun—to stick to your plan long enough for a new action to become habit.

Competition. Nothing like a little friendly competition to keep you engaged. Enroll your co-workers in a "bring your lunch from home" challenge. Or there are many apps—such as Challenge Hound and The Conqueror— that let you pick a certain challenge, such as walking the length of Ireland, in a certain amount of time, and then invite friends and family to join you. As you log your steps each day, you'll see your progress on the map—and see who's ahead and who's behind you. Knowing that your friends can see your progress can be a real motivator.

Gamification. Playing on the rewards theme, you can also turn your new habit into a game. I've seen yoga studios and bookstores create a bingo card designed to get people to practice or read more—each time you complete a specific task on your bingo card (such as "do your three least favorite poses" or "read a graphic novel"), you cross out that square. Get a whole row, or even black out your whole card, and you are entered into a drawing or earn a reward. This is the equivalent of the sticker chart you may have made for your kids when they were learning how to do their chores. Fill up the row, get a prize, and—better yet—build a new habit. You can make a bingo card for yourself, or you and a few friends, and decide on your own rewards, or find some other way to make a game out of your efforts.

Collaboration. The buddy system or having someone you can check in with to report your progress, share your struggles, and brainstorm new solutions can help you stay motivated. Of course, if you want or need to go it alone, that's fine. Again, there is no one-size-fits-all solution.

Professional support. Maybe you need more than a friendly ear and want to consider hiring an expert to help you understand better what makes you tick and guide you in your pursuits, such as a therapist or a coach.

Peer support. You may want to ask friends and family to be part of your support team, check in on you, and listen to how it's going. You can let them know how much advice you'd like to receive from them.

STEP 5: COURSE-CORRECT

When NASA sends a craft into space, they plot a meticulous course to send that ship to a specific destination across millions of miles in a zero-gravity environment. And still, every trip requires a series of course corrections—or, in NASA terms, "trajectory correction maneuvers" (TCMs). Ninety percent of the time, they are course-correcting.

Any journey to ageless aging requires course correction, too. While planning is helpful, you've also got to be flexible. There are any number of reasons you could get sidetracked or fall off the path altogether: a holiday gathering where you end up eating and drinking too much and then feeling too sluggish to exercise, or you catch a virus, or someone you love gets sick and you need to spend time and energy caring for them, or you pull a muscle and can't do your favorite form of exercise for a while. It's not a question of if, but when and what.

Dr. Kopecky put it like this: "You're going to have setbacks. You're going to go backwards. But don't give up. You've got to keep trying." It's so important to accept that these detours are a normal part of life, and that it's equally as important to get right back to mixing your holistic recipe as soon as possible, and to the extent that you are able.

Even DeEtte, the gold medal–winning Senior Games swimmer who is utterly devoted to taking care of herself, told me that while most days she is indeed living in her bliss point, "there are things that keep taking me away from that point." For DeEtte, it might be a church potluck supper that's chock-full of macaroni and cheese and cupcakes, or it might be an upset with a member of her family who isn't supportive of the choices she's made to take better care of herself. But she has learned how to get herself back to that bliss point after every detour.

How? She describes it this way: "I make better decisions, and I lean into the framework that I know works for me." DeEtte's framework includes swimming every morning, eating healthily, not drinking, and volunteering. "I just want that bliss point more than I want the thing that's trying to pull me off track."

I recently had a conversation with a friend of my husband's from high school. She shared with Ken that she had been having hip problems, and he suggested she reach out to me since I had recently overcome crippling hip pain and had a successful double hip replacement. When we spoke, I told her, "I know it's scary, but it's actually really simple to take a few steps to get rid of the pain." I started by sharing the dietary changes I'd made—no gluten, no dairy, and very little sugar—and the exercise routines that helped me. She said, "Oh, that seems so hard. I'd rather live with the pain." We kept talking, drilling down on how the pain affects her on a daily basis, as well as how she sees her life a year from now, five years from now, and ten years from now if she continues to be in pain. Thinking of the long-term consequences of her short-term reluctance helped motivate her to try at least one thing (she's cutting way down on sugar).

When you start connecting the dots on the things you'd have to potentially give up later—like taking that dream trip to Italy, or dancing with your son or grandson at his wedding—it can help you realize that giving up certain foods now is actually a lot less painful than giving up meaningful experiences in the future.

The good news is that all those course corrections will pay off *soon*. I exercise every day not because I want to stay strong enough to keep doing the hiking and traveling I love to do (although that's a good reason) or because I want to keep heart disease at bay (which I do want), but mostly because it helps me be better able to cope with my daily dose of overwhelm. I'm betting you'll experience a similar lift from incorporating ingredients of ageless aging, and be rewarded with more energy, more clarity, and more resilience. Before too long, that feeling of it being hard will recede and you'll feel better—perhaps even better than you've felt in years.

PUTTING IT ALL TOGETHER

Now that you have the big picture of the steps required to make a plan to begin your ageless aging journey, and you've blocked out time to do them, and you've implemented some strategies to make them stick, you're well equipped to start making changes.

If you're looking for a place to start, I suggest following the outline of the book. Start with the basics: fitness, nutrition, and sleep. I suggest fitness as an easy entry point because you will see relatively fast results that will motivate you to keep going. Even if you're already working out, I will give you fitness tips, techniques, and hacks designed for living longer, better. From there, you will learn how to make changes in your food choices. Even small changes in how you eat can make a big difference. Next, I'll explore how you can improve your sleep, which might already be better from regular exercise and smarter food choices. As you begin to integrate these ingredients, you'll notice how they all work together. Those connections can help propel you forward.

Then I'll dive into a challenging but exciting idea: how you can manage your hormones more effectively as you move toward and through menopause, which so many of us struggle with.

Next, I'll discuss how you can optimize your relationship with healthcare—something that, as I discovered while conducting the research for this book, is a little more complicated than I thought. However, it is vital to your well-being. This affects your quality of life as much or more than you ever realized.

Of course, health doesn't stop at the neck. The brain is an essential part of the ageless aging recipe. It's so important for women, who are twice as likely to experience cognitive decline than men, that I've devoted an entire chapter to it.

Building on these basics, I'll then explore how the heart and soul of ageless aging are all about the mind and spirit. I'll suggest action steps you can use to care for your mental and cognitive health, as well as unleash your mind's power to help you grow. I'll also examine the influence of your relationships and sense of purpose on both the quality and quantity of your longer life, and the strong connection between physical/mental health and money. I've learned that finances are a big part of the head trip that can negatively or positively impact women's efforts to age agelessly.

Along the way, I'll describe some of the ingredients you can explore (and where necessary, discuss with your doctor or financial advisor), including new breakthroughs such as the next generation of wearables and at-home diagnostics, cutting-edge approaches to fitness, tools to help protect your cognitive health, and technology-assisted investment strategies.

It's time to get busy—and it's time to get pumped. This is where you start to take your longevity bonus into your own hands.

CHARTING YOUR PATH: WHERE TO BEGIN

If you do one thing: Make your plan now and write it down
Review your Ageless Aging Assessment from Chapter 1, the audit of

your current circumstances Dr. Suzanne Steinbaum suggests in this chapter, and then choose one, two, or at most three things you want to start doing differently today. Write them down on a piece of paper, as this simple act has been shown to improve the odds of success.

If you're already doing a lot to promote ageless aging and are ready to take it to the next level: "Plus" a positive and course-correct a negative

There are two ways to make beneficial changes—build on what's going well, and course-correct the things that aren't. A way to simplify this process is to look at your audit, choose one positive thing and one negative thing, and think about how you can "plus" the positive and course-correct the negative.

Keep it simple but specific and write both your positive and negative down. Your positive may be something like "I exercised this morning," or "I got to spend time with my grandkids yesterday." Then explore if there are ways you can make them even better the next time. For example, could you make it a point to go up a hill on tomorrow's walk? Could you send your grandkids a text and let them know how much you enjoyed being with them?

Don't forget to look at your list of negatives, which might include things like "I didn't sleep well last night" or "My neck feels tight, and it hurts." What can you commit to doing differently today or tonight to help you sleep better? For your aching neck, could you do some stretches before bed, ask your partner or a friend for a massage, or adjust your office setup so you can sit with better posture?

AGELESS AGING HACKS TO CHART YOUR COURSE

Calendar your goals and time commitments

For whatever step you've decided to start with, it's time to get out your calendar and choose dates and times for you to do it. Put technology to good use and also opt to have a reminder sent to you—and make it recurring if you can. In addition to Cassie Holmes's point that claiming the time in your calendar helps you (a) not worry about the other things you could be doing, (b) increase self-efficacy, and (c) boost your feeling of time affluence, there's also science to show that opting to remind yourself helps increase the odds that you'll actually do it.[3]

Fuel your motivation by increasing levels of glutathione

Researchers at the Swiss Federal Institute of Technology have examined a link between antioxidants and motivation—particularly the number one antioxidant for the brain, a protein called glutathione—in both human and animal experiments. Those with higher levels of glutathione in the brain region associated with motivation performed better and more consistently in motivation tasks.[4]

The researchers then tested whether giving a glutathione precursor, N-acetylcysteine (NAC), had a similar performance-enhancing effect on tasks designed to test motivation. The researchers concluded, "Our study represents a proof of principle that dietary N-acetylcysteine can increase brain glutathione levels and facilitate effortful behavior."

You can get NAC through supplements, or by increasing your intake of cysteine—a precursor to NAC that is readily available in high-protein foods including meat, chicken, fish, seafood, eggs, legumes, whole grains, and broccoli.[5]

Part 2

◆

THE HOLISTIC RECIPE FOR AGELESS AGING

4

FITNESS 2.0, THE SILVER BULLET

We used to think that how we aged was already encoded in our genes, fostering a convenient "this is out of my hands" attitude. That myth was busted in 1998 when Dr. John Rowe and Robert Kahn published *Successful Aging*, introducing the landmark findings of the MacArthur Foundation Study of Aging in America. As I mentioned in Chapter 1, the study turned the 70/30 rule on its head and suggested that if there's a silver bullet to turning back the hands of time, it's regular exercise. Two words: *regular* and *exercise*.

Today, we're hearing more and more stories of women in the second half of their lives transforming their health and their lives through fitness. Even if you're never considered yourself athletic, or even that active, it is absolutely possible to be in the best shape of your life at fifty, sixty, seventy, or beyond.

Take Joan McDonald, who reinvented her future at age seventy. Just five foot three and weighing almost two hundred pounds, Joan was on a downward slide, already taking medications for high blood pressure and acid reflux, experiencing painful arthritis and terrible swelling in her ankles, and having difficulty walking up and down stairs. She was both physically and emotionally exhausted and frightened about what might lie ahead.

Joan was able to reinvent herself with the help of her daughter, Michelle, and a support network of like-minded new friends. Michelle, a transformation coach, was so worried about her mother's future that she intervened, explaining to her mom that she was at a pivotal turning point. If she continued on her current path, Joan would likely be taking even more medication, experiencing even more pain and anxiety, and end up even worse off. Her future did not look pretty.

Michelle offered her mom the chance to participate in an online group, the Wonder Women Collective, with other women who were working to take better care of themselves and reinvent their lives. Initially Joan was skeptical, but she decided she had nothing to lose. With the support and guidance of Michelle and the other women in the group, she made a 180-degree change, beginning with simple steps. She renewed her gym membership, bought a food scale and measuring tape, and joined the online group of women who were building exercise into their lives.

Joan's motto was "I don't mind if my changes are slow. I am going to go at my own pace, and this time the changes are going to last for the rest of my life."

Fast-forward to today. At age seventy-four, Joan sees a brighter future than she ever imagined. Not only has she lost more than fifty pounds, she can also navigate the gym with confidence. She says that connecting with other women who are choosing to live a healthier lifestyle is what she enjoys most. Joan is creating a path to ageless aging, which, by the way, she joyfully shares with her 1.4 million Instagram followers (at this writing).

No matter what your relationship to movement has been in the past—whether you've embraced it, or avoided it, or been somewhere in between—moving your body needs to be part of your ageless aging plan.

First, it offers a mind-boggling array of benefits for your body, mind, and relationships. (I'll take you through those in just a moment.) Just as important, when you start to move your body more, you trigger a cascade of positive side effects. You sleep better because you've expended more energy during the day. You feel less stressed and anxious because exercise clears your head. You begin to feel more empowered as your body builds strength and endurance, allowing you to climb stairs or hills without getting out of breath. Regular exercise helps make every other ingredient you add to your ageless aging stone soup that much more doable. And it doesn't take a lot of thought or prep work to implement—as you'll see in this chapter, there are so many meaningful ways to improve your fitness, while also adding richness and good old-fashioned fun to your life.

I believe that once you take a closer look at all the reasons why exercise—and movement in general—is beneficial to every aspect of your ageless aging, you'll be convinced to embrace fitness in new ways.

THE ASTOUNDING BENEFITS OF MOVEMENT

Nearly all longevity experts now agree that regular movement is one of the most effective geroprotective strategies. Why? The human body is designed to move. Our ancestors spent ten to fifteen hours a day involved in vigorous activities as a matter of survival. We have evolved (or perhaps I should say devolved) from active hunters and gatherers into sedentary couch potatoes. Today, most of us sit for hours behind computer screens or in front of the TV. If you've ever had a cast on an arm or a leg, you've seen how that limb lost much of its strength and mobility by the time the cast was removed. That's because your muscles atrophied and your circulation was diminished. The same thing happens if you don't move your body—it will atrophy and cease to function optimally. Movement helps you avoid the deterioration associated with aging, such as joint pain, limited mobility, and loss of flexibility. And the benefits don't end there.

Let's explore the list of all the wonderful things regular movement can do.

- **Lowers biological age.** Dr. Kara Fitzgerald calls movement "an anti-aging elixir that spins the biological clock in reverse." She is the author of *Younger You* and a functional medicine provider/

researcher whose specialty is prescribing specific foods and lifestyle practices to reduce biological aging. A single exercise session has been shown to trigger beneficial changes to your genetic expression—turning bad genes off and turning good genes on.[1] Now imagine how those changes add up when you make movement a consistent part of your life.

- **Reduces risk of cancer.** The International Agency for Research on Cancer posits that 25 percent of all cancers are the result of the health cascades associated with being sedentary. Getting regular movement has been clearly linked to significantly reduced risks of thirteen different types of cancers, including lung, colon, and breast cancer. While even light exercise counts, the more and more intensely you exercise, the more pronounced the reductions in risk are.[2]

- **Lowers risk of stroke.** A 2022 study that followed the daily movements of over 6,700 adults forty-five and older and published in the *Journal of the American Medical Association* found that every hour per week you spend doing light activity—like cleaning house or preparing food—creates a 14 percent reduction in stroke risk.[3] And spending at least 175 minutes per week (that's just shy of three hours per week) in moderate to vigorous activity, such as playing tennis (doubles or singles), walking vigorously, climbing stairs, swimming, or gardening, is associated with a 43 percent reduced risk of stroke. (I love that this study counted more everyday movements and didn't just look at official "exercise.")

- **Reduces risk of type 2 diabetes.** A 2016 meta-analysis of twenty-eight studies (with a total pool of over 1.2 million participants) evaluated the effectiveness of physical activity at lowering the risk of developing type 2 diabetes. The results were clear: the more you exercise, the greater the reduction in risk. If you manage to get 150 minutes per week of moderate exercise (two and a half hours over the course of seven days), your risk is 26 percent lower; at 300 minutes per week (five total hours per week), the risk is 36 percent lower. And spending more hours in motion at a higher intensity was accompanied by a 56 percent reduction in risk compared to people who were inactive.[4]

- **Reduces risk of premature death from heart disease.** Researchers from Harvard's School of Public Health analyzed data collected over thirty years and found that people who exercised 150 minutes a week at a moderate intensity (walking, weight lifting) had a 25 percent lower risk of dying from cardiovascular disease, while those who worked out seventy-five minutes a week at a more vigorous intensity (jogging, cycling, or swimming) saw a reduction in risk of 31 percent.[5]

- **Reduces risk of osteoporosis.** Exercise also strengthens your bones and prevents falls—a double whammy of benefits. On the flip side, the less you move, the more likely you are to lose bone density, which makes you more vulnerable to breaking a bone if you fall. Moving less also makes you stiffer, weaker, and less agile. In a meta-analysis of studies that assessed more than thirty thousand postmenopausal women, those who exercised regularly were significantly less likely to develop osteoporosis than those who didn't. Bones respond to load and impact, so the less weight bearing your bones have to do—and the less impact they receive—the fewer cues they get to grow stronger.[6]

- **Reverses and prevents sarcopenia.** Since muscle is a lot about "use it or lose it," we often lose it as we live longer, because we tend to move less as we get older. Sure, aging itself contributes to loss of muscle mass, but regular exercise helps you maintain and even grow muscle mass. It's important to note that maintaining your muscles as you age also requires upping your protein intake—something we'll cover in the next chapter.

- **Boosts mood.** Movement balances your neurotransmitters, lessens the experience of depression and anxiety, and produces natural painkilling molecules such as endorphins. For me, exercise is as much about impacting my mental and emotional well-being as it is improving my physical health. If I don't exercise, I start to feel down, anxious, and moody. Exercise keeps me feeling alert, positive, energetic, and even-keeled. It's my drug of choice.

- **Improves cognitive function.** Physical movement boosts the function of your entire body, including your brain. According to the Alzheimer's Association, there's a broad body of research that shows that getting more exercise is one of the most powerful lifestyle changes you can make to protect your cognitive function for life. Exercise can increase the size of the hippocampus—the brain region associated with memory that tends to shrink in people with dementia. Specifically, regular movement can lower your risk of developing dementia by 30 percent and developing Alzheimer's by 45 percent.[7]

- We are beginning to understand that a major player in the cognitive benefit of exercise is brain-derived neurotrophic factor (BDNF)—a chemical messenger that cues the brain to form new neurons, lay down new memories and access old memories, learn, access higher-thinking functions, and alleviate depression and anxiety. It's magical stuff—and you just have to move your body to get a dose of it.

Regular movement is also what's known as *hormesis*, or a moderate form of stress that produces a beneficial, adaptive response. In other words, it challenges the body and forces it to grow stronger and become more resilient. It does so by triggering cellular repair processes that, once turned on, continue the rebuilding process beyond the starting point. In addition, physical activity also helps you enjoy higher energy levels, aids digestion, improves liver health, is associated with a rise in high-density lipoprotein (the good kind of cholesterol), and even, according to Harvard Medical School, can make your sex life better.[8] Clearly, it's time to get moving. Or, if you already exercise regularly, add in some different types of movement.

Let's take a look at the major categories of physical activity so you can get some new ideas and, to use a financial analogy, recognize where your movement portfolio may need a little rebalancing.

SIX ESSENTIAL TYPES OF MOVEMENT AND EXERCISE

I've noticed that many women (including me) tend to focus regularly on only one type of movement—maybe it's cardio, Pilates, hiking, or yoga. However, as we live longer, women especially need to do a *combination* of different types of exercise. When I interviewed biomechanist Katy Bowman, founder of Nutritious Movement and the author of numerous books on the benefits of movement, including *Move Your DNA*, she told me to think of movement like food. "You need to have a really well-rounded movement diet that has adequate amounts of movement, as well as a wide variety of movements," she said. "We know when it comes to diet, we need to eat the rainbow. The same is true for movement. We need to move the rainbow."

This may sound like a lot to do, and I know you probably don't have all day to devote to moving your body in a wide variety of ways, but there are ways to combine different forms of physical activity to satisfy multiple movement needs at once. Also, once you get in the habit of moving more and enjoy the added energy, mobility, and vitality it can bring, you might be inspired to find more ways to do more of it.

Let's identify the six main types of physical activity—what it is, why you need it, and how you can assess how well you're doing in each category.

Cardio

Cardiovascular exercise, also known as aerobic exercise, is any rhythmic exercise that gets your heart rate and respiration up and pushes your metabolism into a fat- and calorie-burning zone. Cardio helps strengthen your heart, your lungs, and—if it's high-impact or weight-bearing—your bones.

The easiest, most accessible way to get your cardio is to walk. You've probably heard the advice to get 10,000 steps per day, but in recent years it's come to light that number was popularized because it was easy to remember, not necessarily because it had any evidence to support it. A 2022 study that followed more than six thousand adults who wore fitness trackers over the course of four years lowered the bar for a daily step target to 8,200. That's the magic number where participants unlocked a significantly decreased risk of developing a range of chronic diseases, including obesity, sleep apnea, major depressive disorder, type 2 diabetes, high blood pressure, and gastroesophageal reflex disease (GERD).[9]

A fitness tracker, such as a FitBit, pedometer, or Apple Watch makes it very easy—and addictive—to track how many steps you take in a day. But you don't need a specific device to track your movement. You can grab your iPhone and click on the Health app (the little white icon with a big red heart on it) or your Android device and open the Google Fit app to turn them on. Then you can keep your phone on you during the day and see what your baseline number of steps is—and track what it feels like to walk more.

An important subset of cardio exercise that can boost the impact of your exercise while saving you time is high-intensity interval training (HIIT). A 2017 study in *Cell Metabolism* suggests that HIIT

Ways to Boost the Intensity—and the Benefit—of a Walk

- Incorporate intervals of walking as fast as you can and pumping your arms.
- Walk holding one- or two-pound weights.
- Climb stairs or hills.
- Vary your speed.
- Use walking poles, which turn walking into a full-body workout.
- Listen to up-tempo music, which will naturally increase your pace.
- Walk over uneven terrain, such as a forest floor, grass, or a cobblestone street; though you may need to go more slowly, you will challenge your stabilizing muscles more.

workouts can reverse the signs of aging at the cellular level and boost mitochondrial capacity (remember, mitochondria are the energy factories of your cells). The older you are, the more your mitochondria stand to benefit.[10]

You can turn any workout into a HIIT workout by spending a short amount of time—typically somewhere between thirty and sixty seconds—going as hard as you can, and then resting, typically for slightly less time than you pushed yourself or the same amount of time. If you are walking, you could build in some HIIT by walking as fast as you can and pumping your arms for one minute, then resting for thirty seconds, and repeating that cycle another five times before resuming your normal-paced walk. If you go to a gym, most cardio machines will run you through a HIIT workout if you select it on the machine's dashboard.

And perhaps you've heard of the famous Seven-Minute Workout (if you haven't, a quick Google search is all it takes). It's a HIIT workout that uses bodyweight exercises for a session that combines cardio, intensity, and strength training in one seven-minute session, which is a great hack. Beyond the benefits of regular cardio exercise, HIIT offers specific results, including improved cognition, specifically executive function;[11] burning fat, particularly abdominal fat, which is the most dangerous type of fat, as it emits pro-inflammatory molecules and is associated with greater health risk than fat that is stored around the hips and thighs;[12] and lowering fasting insulin levels.[13] For me, a HIIT workout using weights—which will tick your boxes for cardio, strength, and intensity—is the best fitness bang for your buck.

Types of cardio exercises: Walking, jogging, running, hiking, rowing, bicycling, tennis, pickleball, swimming, dancing, aerobics classes, kickboxing classes, using the cardio machines at the gym.

Strength training

According to Carla Prado, PhD, professor of nutrition at the University of Alberta, "Muscle mass should be looked at as a new vital sign." Prado was the principal author of a 2018 meta-analysis that found having more muscle mass gave women with breast cancer a 60 percent higher survival rate and helped people in the ICU spend less time on ventilators, get out of the ICU faster, and enjoy improved quality of life and survival rates.[14] Basically, having more muscle (aka lean body mass) is like taking out an umbrella insurance policy on your health.

Strength training is not about building bulk or getting "cut." You can build lean, long muscles by using less weight with more repetitions. Strength training helps you stay healthier longer to continue doing all the things you enjoy in life—as well as giving you that nice, toned look.

But maintaining muscle mass is something you have to consciously do. Conventional wisdom has it that after we turn forty, we lose about 8 percent of our muscle tissue every decade. That's sarcopenia. "I don't care if you're an Olympian, we're all going to end up losing some lean body mass. That means as you age, strength training becomes more and more important for a whole host of reasons, including to just be able to survive," Dr. Pamela Peeke, assistant professor of medicine at the University of Maryland School of Medicine, adjunct senior scientist at the National Institutes of Health, and bestselling author of *Body for Life for Women* and *Fight Fat After Forty*, told me. "The challenge is, it's also harder to put muscle on once you're past the age of sixty."

If you don't manage to maintain muscle as you age, "you start getting way too close to not having enough to be independent and functional, and that's not a good place to be," Peeke warned, adding, "If you fall down on the floor, do you see a front-end loader showing up to pick you up? Who's going to reach for that thing that you need, and pull it down?" Most of us share the goal of remaining self-sufficient, but there's even more to it than maintaining independence.[15] Other specific benefits of strength training include:

- **Increased strength.** When you lift weights, your muscles get the cue to build back stronger.
- **More energy.** The more your muscles are in the state of pushing, pulling, or holding weight, the more adenosine triphosphate

(ATP)—the form of energy that fuels most bodily processes—
you burn through. That depletion of ATP turns on a chemical
response to not just replenish it, but also trigger changes to your
gene expression that support burning excess sugar and fat for fuel.

- **Higher metabolism.** Muscle tissue requires more energy to
  maintain, which means that as you increase your muscle mass,
  your metabolism also rises—great for weight management.
- **Stronger bones.** Since muscles pull on bones, and bones respond
  to that pressure by growing stronger and denser, when we build
  muscle, we also build bone density.

Research has demonstrated that it only takes two resistance training sessions per week to reverse the muscle loss caused by age-related
changes.[16] "So I don't care how old you are," Peeke said. "Start right
now to build more lean muscle mass."

Types of exercise that improve strength: Lifting weights, doing bodyweight exercises (such as squats, planks, and push-ups), using resistance
machines at the gym, isometric contractions (holding a certain position
for a minute or more), HIIT using weights or resistance bands, yoga,
Pilates, tai chi, and martial arts.

Balance

It's never too late to improve your balance, but you don't want to wait
until you feel wobbly to strengthen it. Balance is vital for many reasons—of
course, it helps prevent falls, but it also helps you with daily life, as there
are many times when all your weight is on just one leg: getting out of a car,
taking a step, climbing a stair. Balance is also closely linked with mobility
and agility. If you feel off-balance or shaky on your feet, you'll become
more and more likely to avoid different types of movement, and that's
not the direction we want to be heading on our ageless aging journey.

While strength training will help you have the strength to maintain your balance, you also need fluidity. Chungliang "Al" Huang,
internationally acclaimed tai chi master and educator and one of the

most joyful people I've ever met (he officiated when my husband, Ken, and I renewed our vows in Big Sur, California), says tai chi is one of the best kinds of movement for women as they live longer, precisely because it helps them develop and maintain balance and fluidity. "Tai chi movement is a joyful way of expressing yourself," he told me. It's a series of standing postures and hand gestures that flow from one into the other like a slow-motion dance that builds strength and balance throughout your whole embodiment—mind, body, and spirit. "Tai chi is so important because it allows your energy, your breathing, your whole musculature to not be blocked," Huang said. And when your energy is flowing throughout your body without impediment, "you're more at ease; you just feel better; even your facial expression will change. You project youth even though you're getting older."

Tai chi has an impressive body of research to suggest that it helps reduce the likelihood of falling—as well as reducing back pain and pain from osteoarthritis, improving cognitive function, and raising quality of life.[17]

You can take tai chi as a class—look at your local gym, library, or community center, or at a dedicated tai chi center—and, once you've learned some of the forms, you can practice on your own at home, or in a park, which is where you'll see people well into their elder years practicing it if you visit China. Huang advises that you look for a teacher who is clearly enjoying themselves: "If the teacher smiles and the class looks like they're having fun, that's a good class," he said. "But if the teacher looks glum and the participants look stiff and scared, stay away."

Types of exercise that improve balance: Tai chi, yoga, Pilates, and dancing, which all put you in positions where your weight is on one leg and improve core strength and flexibility. And the balance that biking requires may make it even more impactful at building your balance when your feet are on the ground. In addition, just making it a point to spend some time throughout your day with all your weight supported by one leg and then the other will improve your balance, too.

Quick Longevity Assessment #1: Flamingo Test

Being able to maintain your balance is essential to longevity. In fact, a study published in the *British Journal of Sports Medicine* asked people ages fifty-one to seventy-five to remove their shoes and socks and balance on one leg for ten seconds. Twenty percent of the participants couldn't do it— and seven years later, those who couldn't do it were 84 percent more likely to have died than those who could.[18]

Can you stand on one leg like a flamingo for ten seconds? Try it! Stand tall with your head high and arms at your sides, transfer your weight to one foot, and then lift the other foot into the air. Be sure to do this standing close to a wall, chair, or table in case you lose your balance. Count how many seconds you can stay upright. Then repeat on the other leg. Don't panic if you can't stand on one leg even for a few seconds. If you do this exercise daily, you will improve your balance dramatically and may add years of health to your life.

Functional movement and posture

Functional movement, otherwise known as mobility training, is a collection of exercises designed to help you do anything you need to do during the course of a normal day more efficiently—such as bending, twisting, lifting, pushing, pulling, sitting, standing, putting on your shoes, and getting into and out of your car. You may think these are no-brainer things that you don't need to practice, but it's generally doing these everyday things where we get injured; both because real life is random (you have to pick up the heavy box from your porch and carry it into your home while holding the door open, for example) and because these are the movements we do every day without much thought to *how* we're doing them.

Look for classes at your local gym with "functional" in the title. Or, if your doctor has ever told you that you need physical therapy, get yourself to PT. Chances are it will be covered by medical insurance. Functional fitness tends to include bodyweight strength movements such as squats and deadlifts, so it can fulfill some of your need for strength training, too.

Postural alignment is responsible for so many things—muscle pain and tightness, wear and tear on your joints, even your digestion and pelvic health. If you constantly slouch, not only will you look elderly, but your abdominal organs will begin to compress, impairing their function and causing even more weight to be borne by your pelvic floor. While yoga, Pilates, and tai chi can help you build core strength and find proper alignment to improve posture, the way you hold your body during your daily life also has a huge impact on your overall posture, impacting your ageless aging. Here are two simple postural adjustments:

- **Head ramping.** This brings your ears over your shoulder and reduces strain on your neck and upper back muscles. To do it, adjust your chin position so that it is parallel to the ground, then glide the back of your head back so that your ears are over your shoulders. Repeat as necessary.
- **Wearable posture support.** There are many different wearable devices that help to remind you to keep your spine straight. (If you're interested in a brace that provides more support to the spine, check with your doctor first as the body can become overly dependent on the device to do the work of holding your spine in alignment.) My daughter-in-law, FeyFey, uses the Go2 wearable posture trainer and finds it useful. Another company that makes an electronic posture sensor is Amszke. "The real benefit of these devices is that they bring your awareness to your posture and that alone can reduce pain and increase confidence," says Neel Anand, MD, a professor of orthopedic surgery and the director of spine trauma at Cedars-Sinai Spine Center in Los Angeles.[19]

Types of exercise to strengthen this aspect of fitness: Yoga, Pilates, and tai chi all build body awareness, strength, and flexibility—a combination that really helps those everyday movements happen more gracefully. Bodyweight strength training and functional fitness classes also help; physical therapy can help identify and address any muscle imbalances or postural misalignments that may be impeding your body's function.

Quick Longevity Assessment #2: Sit/Rise Test

Here's another baseline movement test to access overall health and potential longevity, as it measures lower body strength, mobility, and flexibility. This simple test requires you to start from standing, sit down on the floor, and then stand back up again. It's helpful to cross one leg behind the other before you begin your descent, so that you can end in a cross-legged position, and to be near a chair or coffee table you can lean on for assistance if your balance wavers. When you're going down to the floor, you subtract 1 point from a total of 10 for every time you have to bring a body part to the floor besides your butt—a knee, an elbow, a forearm. You also subtract a point from bringing a hand or forearm to your knee, or the side of your leg, or the chair or coffee table for support. Then do the same scorekeeping on the way back up, subtracting a point for each touch from a beginning score of five. So the top score is 10, and the lowest is 0.

Lower scores have been associated with higher mortality; every point increase in score is linked to a 21 percent improvement in survival rates. If you've had hip or knee replacement, or have a mobility challenge such as arthritis or chronic pain, this test is less applicable. And, remember, you can improve your score with practice, so don't lose hope if you start with a low score.

Sit/rise test score guide

0–3	Unhealthy
4–7	Compromised health
8–10	Good health

Flexibility

Stretching helps your muscles elongate and relax as well as grow stronger. Tight muscles are weak muscles. Stretching increases the flow of blood to your muscles, improves the way synovial fluid moves in your joints to keep the joints lubricated, and helps improve your range of motion. Stretching also promotes relaxation—it has been shown to boost levels of serotonin, the neurotransmitter that plays such an important role in mood, and is believed to trigger the release of endorphins—natural painkillers and mood boosters.[20]

Best of all, stretching is something you can easily incorporate into your daily life by taking stretch breaks throughout the day, or building a new habit of doing some stretches while watching TV or as part of your wind-down routine before bed.

Stretching also helps keep your fascia healthy. Fascia is a type of tissue that encases your muscles, sort of like plastic wrap, and while we are still learning about its many functions, fascia is supposed to easily glide over our muscles. But with our stressful, sedentary lives, it's common for fascia to get dried out and contract in what's known as fascial adhesion, where it's almost like the muscle fibers and fascia become glued together, creating internal scar tissue that impedes movement.

I admit that I have tipped the scales more toward cardio and strength and, although I love my weekly Pilates class, have otherwise neglected flexibility. I recently got a myofascial release treatment— during the treatment I thought nothing much was happening, but I got my best night's sleep of the year the night after and felt much more fluid throughout my body. It's something I plan to incorporate into my regular self-care routine—and luckily you don't always have to visit a practitioner to release your fascia. Rolling on a foam roller, tennis balls, or self-massage balls can help loosen tight muscles and fascial adhesions, too.

Types of exercise to strengthen this area of fitness: Stretching, yoga (especially restorative yoga and yin yoga, which holds restorative poses for longer times and is designed to bring more flexibility into connective tissue), Pilates, tai chi, barre.

Relaxation and Breathing

As important as building strength and cardio endurance are, they are only one side of the coin. We also need to support and bolster our ability to relax, because it is only when we are experiencing true physiological relaxation (known as the relaxation response) that we can rest, digest, listen to our inner wisdom, and gently heal. To be resilient means not only that you are strong in the face of adversity, but also that you can integrate the lessons adversity taught you and come back stronger— and you need the benefits of relaxation to be able to bounce back. As Dr. Peeke told me, "You have to take care of your mental fitness as well as your physical fitness."

Of course, a well-studied approach to promoting relaxation is meditation—something I'll cover more in Chapter 9. But even taking a few minutes to focus on your breathing, either before or after your movement practice, or as a mental break at some point in your day, can invite more relaxation into your life.

It can be as simple as finding an empty conference room and putting your head down for five minutes or staring out the window at the horizon or the sky while paying attention to each breath as it happens. When Dr. Peeke was working overnight shifts at the hospital, she'd go up to the roof of the hospital for ten minutes and take in the stars.

Breathing is something we do automatically all the time, but when we're anxious or stressed, we may be holding our breath or taking shallower breaths. Deep breathing is a great form of relaxation. Every night before we go to sleep, my husband and I have made a ritual of doing a two-minute breathing exercise that's available at low cost on an app called Breathwrk. To be sure, there are numerous apps that are available for this and many other purposes. It's like magic for us. It relaxes the body and mind so that we fall asleep within minutes.

There is no shortage of healing modalities that can help you access that relaxed state, including massage, acupuncture, autogenic training, HeartMath, craniosacral therapy, and more. Tools like percussive massage guns are also a very effective and fun way to either self-massage or massage with a partner.

Relaxing Breathing Techniques

Bringing awareness and intention to the way you are breathing can help you initiate the relaxation response wherever you are. Try these and see what works best for you.

Box breathing. Inhale for a count of four, hold for four, exhale for four, and hold your breath out for four before starting the cycle again. Repeat for eight to ten cycles.

Extended exhale. Inhale for a count of three, exhale for a count of six. To expel this much air, you have to really engage your diaphragm muscle, which can get locked when you are stressed. Getting it moving again sends the all-clear signal to your nervous system. This breath is great to do while lying in bed to help you relax into sleep.

Inhale, exhale, pause. Breathe normally, but after each exhale pause just a beat or two. This is a great thing to do in everyday stressful situations, like a dentist's visit or sitting in traffic. It gives your mind a focus and your consciousness a chance to rest.

Types of exercise to strengthen this area of fitness: Yoga (especially restorative or yin yoga), tai chi, stretching, breathing exercises, massage, acupuncture, autogenic training, HeartMath, finding meaningful ways to build mental rest into your day.

SITTING IS THE NEW SMOKING

Hippocrates wrote in 400 BC, "All parts of the body have a function, if used in moderation. But if unused and left to idle, they become liable to disease, defective in growth and age quickly." As beneficial as the different forms of physical fitness are, the simple truth is that we need to move more and in more ways. This is something we don't typically do. Most of us have a major movement deficiency—in large part because as a society, we have transitioned from a highly active lifestyle to a primarily sedentary one.

Sitting for more than six hours every day and being less active is associated with a 94 percent increase in the risk of premature death from any cause in women.[21] We simply have to break out of the chair and the couch—it's killing us not to.

Ways to Interrupt Sitting at Work

If you have a desk job, it may seem impossible to build more movement into your day. But there *are* ways to make sitting less harmful. They include:

Sitting on an exercise ball. Replacing your office chair with one of the big stability balls you might use to help you stretch at the gym requires you to engage your core muscles and has been found to boost your overall daily expenditure of calories—which can ward off weight gain over time.[22] There are also cushions with a curved base so that you have to use your core stabilizing muscles as you sit—I have one and love it. It's a little more stable than an exercise ball, so I'm not worried about completely rolling off.

Standing breaks. My husband and I joke that when we have something we need to write that it's time to "get our butts in the chair," but just because you have work to do, that doesn't mean you have to remain glued to your seat. Building a new habit of periodically standing up and stretching during the workday can help by bringing down glucose levels, burning a few extra calories, and just giving your body some of the movement it craves. Setting a timer to remind yourself to stand up every twenty minutes has been shown to improve blood pressure and provide a small, but still helpful, reduction in all-cause mortality risk. It also reduces blood glucose levels after eating in middle-aged adults.[23] Of course, you can also use a standing or treadmill desk for some or all of your workday; it's an investment of money and space, but one that will help you reap the benefits of movement without feeling like you need to find more time in your day to go exercise.

Walking breaks. Taking breaks to do a little light-intensity walking is even better than standing, as it has been shown to bring down blood glucose levels and insulin levels.[24] Although we have an idea that in order to be a good worker we need to sit still and focus, taking a break between tasks to get up and move a bit will refresh your mind as well as benefit your body.

As much as I love exercise, consciously adding all kinds of movement into our daily life is also essential. To make your day more movement-rich, do some of your errands on foot. Take the stairs instead of the escalator. Set up a standing workstation where you can answer emails or do Zoom calls. Sit on the floor and do some stretches while you watch Netflix in the evening.

There's a scientific term for this type of movement: non-exercise activity thermogenesis (NEAT). It refers to the calories you burn doing anything that is *not* sleeping, eating, or official exercise—basically, all the movements required as part of daily living, such as washing dishes, sweeping, walking to the car, walking the aisles at the store, carrying groceries, climbing stairs, folding laundry. They all add up and have been shown to contribute to some impressive health benefits, including increasing insulin sensitivity, lowering blood pressure, burning extra calories, increasing good cholesterol, and reducing risk of all-cause mortality.[25]

It's time we consider rethinking our relationship to chores—instead of seeing them as something that takes us away from being produc-tive that we need to minimize, they can be an opportunity for more movement. "Chores are an easy source of bending over, picking things up, keeping your joints mobile, keeping your muscles strong, burning calories," Bowman says. As a bonus, reframing the way you think about chores could improve your relationship with your partner or others in your house—since you won't see doing the dishes as the hot potato that you don't want to catch, but rather think of it as another opportunity to sneak movement into your day. If you need more convincing to get pumped about errands and chores, consider that NEAT movements can result in burning up to 2,000 extra calories a day.[26]

FIND YOUR MOTIVATION

The more you can get excited about moving more on multiple planes of existence, the stronger and more lasting your motivation will be. Try some of these emotional and mental motivations to help you get—and stay—moving.

- **Do it for the joy of it.** When I spoke with Chungliang Al Huang about tai chi, he spelled it out so clearly when he said, "The joyfulness is what makes movement good for you." Do what you can to make movement fun—take a class with a friend or partner, listen to music, go for a walk in a beautiful place that uplifts you. Let it feel like play, not another thing on your to-do list.
- **Embrace being a beginner.** I've seen some people in my life block themselves from the joy of going dancing or taking a hike because they feel like they can't do it well. Remember, it's okay to be a beginner. It helps you have what Buddhists call *beginner's mind*—a refreshing lack of expectation and a natural curiosity.
- **Get comfortable with feeling uncomfortable.** "Instead of falling prey to inertia and the desire to stay comfortable on the couch, I want women to wake up and say, 'I'm willing to get uncomfortable. Bring it on!'" Dr. Peeke says.
- **Establish your baseline.** Dr. Peeke suggests, and I agree, that it's absolutely worth the money if you can afford it to hire a certified personal trainer for a fitness assessment—a test of your balance, flexibility, endurance, and strength. She calls it a reality check, and counsels that you "park your ego at the door, because it's

going to be very humbling." But that objective information is going to be motivating, and it's going to give you a "before" snapshot that you can use to measure your progress.

- **Manage your own expectations.** When I spoke with Colin Milner, CEO of the International Council on Active Aging and founder of the active-aging industry in North America, about the biggest challenges to getting older adults to embrace more physical activity, he said two things, and they're both mindset hacks: "Number one is building an identity that says 'I *can* do this' instead of 'I can't.'" The second thing Milner shared is that you can't expect to snap your fingers and automatically become a super-mover. "It took you a certain amount of time to get weaker, so it's going to take you a certain amount of time to get stronger." So, take your increase in fitness in small increments. Aim to get a little better, celebrate your wins, and know that setbacks are just part of the path.

- **Find ways to stack.** Bowman introduced me to the idea of stacking, which is taking care of multiple needs in one action. (It's different from multitasking, which technically is switching rapidly from one task to the other, although it may seem like you're doing two things at once.) Here are some examples as it relates to movement:
  - Walking in the woods with a friend takes care of cardio, time in nature, and friend time.
  - Yoga, Pilates, or tai chi takes care of strength, flexibility, balance, and relaxation in one exercise session.
  - A HIIT workout that uses weights combines cardio, intensity, and strength training.
  - Cleaning the house for thirty minutes is functional exercise, cardio (especially if you are sweeping, vacuuming, or scrubbing), and gets you a clean house. It can also be meditative.
  - Going out dancing is cardio, balance, and social time. It's also joyful.

IF MOVEMENT IS A CHALLENGE

There's often a subconscious expectation that as we get older, we're *supposed* to be able to do less. Katy Bowman reminds us, "You don't have an old body. You do have an accumulation of old habits that prevent you from moving." It's common to have fears of pushing yourself physically, but as Bowman says, "Habits can be changed, and your body will respond to a more movement-rich diet."

However, you may very well have a condition or injury that causes pain or impedes movement for you. The challenge is to focus on what you *can* do, and build on that, rather than get derailed by what you can't do.

Physical activity has been shown to reduce the experience of pain, likely because exercise can produce endorphins, which are nature's painkillers. Getting stronger and improving your range of motion can, in fact, reduce your pain, allowing you to move more.

There are nearly always ways to be more physically active. Resistance machines at the gym can help you build strength with low impact. Chair yoga can help stretch muscles. Pilates can help you strengthen and stretch muscles while adding balance. (Pilates was originally designed by Joseph Pilates when he was serving as a nurse in World War I. He attached springs to a hospital bed so that patients could do some stretching and strengthening to help their recovery. This concept later was translated into the Pilates Reformer. When he moved to America, professional dancers became devoted to Pilates as a way to recover from injuries.) I started doing Pilates to strengthen my ACL after a ski injury. I love it so much that I'm still doing it nearly thirty years later.

"No matter what issues in the tissues you're facing, the prescription is always to move more," Bowman reminds us. "You need to prioritize movement more now than you ever have in your life, because it is the biggest investment in your current and future health you can make."

CUTTING-EDGE APPROACHES TO FITNESS

Throughout the rest of the book, I'll include a look at the newest tools and tactics to take care of each aspect of ageless aging, as well as what's still in development. Here's what's newish in the fitness world.

- **Osteogenic machines.** This is an approach to building bone density, what scientists call *osteogenesis*, quickly and efficiently, and it also increases muscle mass. Osteogenic machines load your bones without impact, using fitness machines that are similar in look to the resistance machines you'd see at a gym. You only need to perform one doable movement for about a minute to get the stimulation to your nervous system that cues your bones to get stronger—a process that takes about ten total active minutes a week. Because you have to visit a facility that has the machines, it can be pricey, but it's efficient—osteogenic machines have been shown to result in a 7 to 14 percent increase in bone density over a duration of six months to a year.[27] My sister-in-law, Linda, was diagnosed with osteopenia, and her doctor suggested that she give it a try to prevent osteoporosis. After several months, she's seen great improvement in her bone density. At this writing, there are a few different companies that offer access to these osteogenic machines—one is OsteoStrong and another is bStrong4Life. However, my guess is that local fitness clubs throughout the country will start offering these as demand grows.
- **Electromyostimulation (EMS).** EMS devices are popping up at local medical spas all over the country. They can engage your muscles in deep contractions without actually activating (or stressing) your central nervous system, joints, or tendons. Again, you need to visit a facility that has EMS machines. They will have you wear a vest and a series of straps around your major muscle groups (such as your glutes, quads, biceps) that will deliver electronic pulses to your muscles while you perform a simple, quick workout.

While you do have to do some exercise with EMS, the electric stimulation maximizes the muscular benefit while minimizing the time. It's also used to strengthen the pelvic floor, which can help with incontinence. A 2020 randomized controlled trial found that women ages fifty-five through sixty-nine who used EMS during a ten-week aerobic and strength-training program experienced greater leg strength, agility, and cardiovascular endurance than women who performed the same program without the EMS equipment.[28] Women of all ages are experimenting with EMS for aesthetic reasons as well, since it builds muscle tone exactly where you want it far faster than traditional exercise. Exercise franchises that focus on EMS include Manduu, Impulse Fitness, and ReBalance, although some gyms, training facilities, physical therapy offices, and medical spas have the equipment, too.

- **Oxygen therapy.** There are three types of oxygen therapy— hyperbaric chambers, exercise with oxygen therapy (EWOT), and contrast oxygen therapy. Hyperbaric chambers require you to rest in a high-pressure environment, either a specially pressurized room or a tube (shaped like a tanning bed), and the extra air pressure naturally forces more oxygen into your lungs. It is a restorative practice, used by athletes to speed recovery time and by doctors as a treatment for such conditions as decompression sickness and carbon monoxide poisoning or to speed wound healing. EWOT and contrast oxygen therapy, on the other hand, require you to exercise while wearing an oxygen mask. Where pressure works to deliver oxygen to your cells with hyperbaric chambers, with EWOT and contrast oxygen therapy the pumping of your heart and increased respiration that happen when you exercise are what usher oxygen more deeply into your respiratory system, your circulatory system, and, ultimately, your cells. EWOT keeps the oxygen levels constant, while contrast oxygen therapy alternates between giving air that has a low concentration of oxygen and air that has a high concentration of oxygen. For both, the suggested frequency is sessions of about fifteen minutes a few times a week. The changes in oxygen levels are believed to cause your smallest blood vessels and capillaries to open more widely and increase oxygen delivery throughout the body, including to the brain (some functional neurology centers use contrast oxygen therapy to help enhance cognitive health and function). You need to visit a facility to use a hyperbaric chamber, and sessions can be expensive (about $75 per hour). You can buy an EWOT or a contrast oxygen therapy setup for your home (through ewot .com or live02.com), although you probably want to try it out at a facility with trained providers first to learn how to use it properly and see if it's for you, as it is an investment.

- **Advanced apparel to supercharge your workout.** Today there are more and more options for exercise clothing with specific health benefits. For example, wearing compression leggings during your workout may help with circulation, decrease soreness, and promote recovery—just search online for "compression leggings" and you'll see a wide array of options. Some leggings even have microbeads woven into the fabric to mimic the effects of a lymphatic drainage massage while you move—the lymphatic system is the waste removal and immune cell delivery system of the body, and it requires movement or manual stimulation for the lymph to flow. I own a pair of MicroPerle compression tights from the company Elastique (the tights retail for $197, although the company has periodic sales) and I do feel more energized when I wear them. Other options include socks woven with NASA-inspired nanoparticles that combine with your own body heat to produce infrared energy, which has been shown to boost circulation and reduce pain. And since sore, aching feet will kill a workout before it even begins, infrared-producing socks may help you move more and get more benefits from that movement. They are available from trueenergysocks.com and are much less of an investment at $19.99 for a three-pack.

There's also a whole emerging category of what's called biometric apparel—shirts that can track your heart rate, heart rate variability (how quickly your heart rate recovers after exertion, widely considered to be a marker of overall health), and even the exertion level of different muscles. Two biometric apparel companies to check out are Athos and Hexoskin.

- **Virtual-reality fitness.** Virtual reality is now being used to help people recover physical function after a stroke, and it can also provide a fun, immersive way to get a variety of workouts in your own home. You need a VR device, such as Meta Quest, and then you'll need to purchase an app to use with that device. You could try boxing, dancing, or high-intensity interval workouts. They have the added benefit of making you feel as if you are working out in a beautiful, exotic location. Some apps are intended to make the workout on your stationary bike, rowing machine, or elliptical machine much more visually compelling and fun. The Meta Quest is an investment—about $400—but once you have it, different apps are about $20 each. One note of caution: Because you're wearing a headset that completely covers your eyes, it's best to have a wide-open room to use your VR headset in, or at least a friend or family member nearby to make sure that you aren't crashing into the furniture or walls.

- **The Vasper System.** Vasper is a workout system that combines compression, cryotherapy, and HIIT and is used by professional athletes, NASA astronauts, elite military squadrons, and celebrities. It's starting to become available to the general public, typically at high-end fitness facilities or functional medicine centers. Dr. Beth McDougall of CLEAR Center of Health and Jyzen Labs, a bio-optimization and functional medicine center in Mill Valley, California, believes they will be available at many gyms and fitness centers in the next five to ten years. The Vasper looks like a high-tech recumbent bike but adds compression straps for your upper arms and upper thighs that restrict blood flow to cool the surface of your skin. "When you are exercising with compression, you build the lactic acid up in the muscles faster and that triggers growth hormone release and reduces inflammatory stress hormones," Dr. McDougall explained to me. "So, in a twenty-one-minute workout you get the benefits of an aerobic [cardio] and anaerobic [strength training and HIIT] workout that also minimizes soreness after the workout." Dr. McDougall says the Vasper is a great tool for people across the fitness spectrum—from those who aren't in shape at all to professional athletes.

FITNESS 2.0: WHERE TO BEGIN

If you do one thing: Start with joy

Do the form of movement you love the most—and commit to doing it regularly. Starting with joy helps you feel more energized. Then you can look to add in a new activity that prioritizes a different—or a few different—categories of fitness.

If you're a total beginner: Aim to walk every day for thirty minutes

Even if you have to start with five or ten minutes and work your way up from there, it's the best way to get started. Once you get up to thirty minutes, it can cut your chances of dying prematurely from heart disease in half. Do it with a friend to get the benefit of socializing and making the time go by faster. Walking indoors, such as at a mall or on a treadmill, counts too, although walking outside gets you natural light and fresh air in addition to movement.

If you already exercise regularly and are ready to take it to the next level: Try something new

If you're a runner, start strength training. If you mostly do low- or moderate-intensity exercise, add one or two HIIT sessions to your weekly routine. If you do mostly cardio, try some restorative yoga. And if you already do a wide variety of movements, learn something new—rock climbing, tango dancing, or pickleball. You'll find more joy and build on your healthy habits with a beginner's mind.

AGELESS AGING HACKS TO MOVE MORE AND BETTER

Optimize *when* you work out

It's not just what you do, but when you do it that matters. Data from a 2022 study with 86,657 male and female participants demonstrated that those who exercised between 8 and 11 a.m. had the lowest risk of coronary heart disease and stroke, and women appeared to benefit even more than men. Research suggests you may boost the fat-burning benefits of exercising in the morning even further by exercising in a fasting state. On the other hand, exercising in the evening, between 7 p.m. and 10 p.m., can disrupt your circadian rhythm (something you'll learn more about in Chapter 7), which is associated with the dysregulation of the neurological, psychiatric, metabolic, cardiovascular, and immunological systems. Of course, that doesn't mean you should skip exercise if you only have time to do it in the afternoons or evenings—some is always better than none.[29]

Pick up the pace of your exercise just three minutes a day
to live longer

Did you know that walking speed is an accurate predictor of longevity? According to a 2019 study, adults with a slower walking gait showed accelerated signs of aging such as cognitive decline and facial aging, compared to their counterparts with a faster walking speed.[30] Another 2022 study shows that picking up the pace of your daily tasks—like race-walking to the bus stop or running up the stairs—just three minutes a day could help you live longer.[31]

Set up your home for more movement

A great way to integrate more movement into your life is to make it easy to do in your home. Install a chin-up bar in your home and you can hang from it a few times a day and get the upper-body-strengthening, chest-opening, and spine-lengthening benefits of hanging in only thirty seconds at a time. Or dust off that basketball hoop you bought for the kids so you can shoot some hoops. Buy a balance board that you leave out in the living room and try to balance during commercial breaks. I keep a balance board near my desk and use it to take breaks. Set out your exercise equipment so that you see it and it will beckon you throughout the day.

Try isometric contractions

Hold a one- or two-pound weight in each hand and stand with your arms out in a T for one minute a few times a week (or a few times a day). This form of strength training is known as isometric contraction training, which my trainer, Nikki Chrysostomou, who is a certified Pilates teacher and osteopath in training, tells me is key for human movement. "In an isometric contraction exercise, the length of the muscle stays the same, which creates long, lean muscle tone, strength, joint stability, and support for your whole body," she says. To make this an exercise for your lower body, too, Chrysostomou suggests coming into a squat with your back resting against the wall while holding the weights with your arms in a T for one minute. Trust me, it works.

Stop outsourcing some of your physical labor

Put your groceries in a basket that you have to carry around rather than a shopping cart that carries the load for you. Rake your own leaves instead of hiring someone with a leaf blower. Hang your laundry out to dry instead of always using the dryer. Get out your nutcracker and shell your own nuts (a great workout for your hands and your grip strength). Find ways to make movement a bigger part of your daily experience.

5

FOOD IS FUEL, FOOD IS MEDICINE, FOOD IS PLEASURE

Once you've begun integrating more movement into your life, it's time to look at the next ingredient in our holistic recipe to increase healthspan, brainspan, and lifespan: food. This includes the "why, what, and when" of eating—why we eat, what to eat, what *not* to eat, how much to eat, and when you should eat.

"Nutrition is the number-one risk factor now for early death and early disease in this country—in the world, for that matter—because we're eating so poorly," Stephen Kopecky, MD, the Mayo Clinic cardiologist you first met in Chapter 1, told me. In fact, he explained that less than 1 percent of adults eat healthily, as per the USDA, mainly because of sugary beverages (sodas, juices, energy drinks, sweetened tea and coffee drinks) and ultra-processed foods, which are also typically loaded with sugar and low in nutrients.

If that doesn't convince you of the importance of food, here's what longevity pioneer Dr. Valter Longo, director of the Longevity Institute at the University of Southern California and author of *The Longevity Diet*, told me: "It is hard to think of anything more powerful than food in determining whether someone is going to make it to a hundred or die before fifty." Today, 70 percent of the world's chronic diseases are due to poor diet. "We already know that type 2 diabetes—one of the most common diseases in the world—is an invention of a modern diet," Dr. Longo says, and just as the modern diet invented type 2 diabetes, changing what you eat can help heal it. "Eating the correct foods . . . can provide the least costly way to take care of a lot of health problems and can be key to a longer and healthier life."[1]

With all the diets floating around and the marketing claims behind the vast array of packaged foods that line grocery store shelves, there's a ton of confusing and conflicting information to wade through. And the importance of getting it right is huge. What we eat directly affects our body, brain, and emotional and spiritual well-being.

Luckily understanding what to eat is not as complicated as it can often feel.

In his book *The Omnivore's Dilemma,* author and journalist Michael Pollan said it simply and best: "Eat real food. Not too much. Mostly plants." And by real food he means food in its whole form, not processed, not from a factory.

I love the relevance of this advice and try to abide by it daily. That being said, a little more specificity can be helpful, particularly when it comes to what, what not, and when to eat. Let's start with what you should eat.

After talking with a wide array of nutrition specialists and researchers, I've distilled the answer into three helpful principles of my own.

- **Prioritize colorful foods.** I'm talking naturally colorful, not blue yogurt or rainbow sprinkle cake.
- **Use simple swaps to upgrade your other food choices.** Replace bad fats with good ones, refined carbs with whole grains, processed foods with real ones, animal proteins with fish and vegetable proteins.
- **Save the less healthy stuff for special occasions.** You don't have to forgo your favorite treats forever. But they need to be the exception, not the rule.

You'll notice that this isn't about cutting out large food groups. It's about adding more of the good stuff, first and foremost, and then knowing which foods you really need to eliminate or relegate to occasional treats.

As Dr. Suzanne Steinbaum, the New York City cardiologist you first met in Chapter 2, told me, "I always tell patients, don't eat crap. You don't have to be obsessive, you just eat mostly vegetarian, and don't eat the bad stuff." Steinbaum does admit that it's not as easy as it is simple. "Getting your diet to that point can be a challenge, but once you've got it down, you don't have to make a big deal over that part of your life."

There are of course times when you need more than fine-tuning. If you're facing any serious disease or chronic condition, food can be more than fuel—it can be medicine. Later in this chapter, I'll cover the eating patterns that through clinical trials and scientific evidence demonstrate their power to prevent or, in some instances, even reverse disease.

There's also another essential role of food in our lives—it's an important source of pleasure. Eating is a chance to engage your senses, savor life, relax around the dinner table, and share time with friends and family. The tastes and smells of food provide sensory gratification and can even convey emotional messages of nurturing and love. I hope that by distilling the basics of dietary choices and empowering you with the knowledge of what foods help promote ageless aging, you will find a way of eating that is pleasurable *and* helps keep you healthy, joyful, and long-lived.

THE "WHY" FOR CHANGING YOUR EATING CHOICES

Before we get into what to eat, let's pause for just a moment to dive deeper into why you want to make dietary change part of your ageless aging recipe. Just as we discussed in the fitness chapter, if you know why you're doing something, you're much more likely to stick to your plan. And when it comes to choosing an eating pattern, knowing your goals can help steer your choices.

Of course, you may have a specific appearance-related goal, such as fitting into a certain pair of jeans or looking great at an upcoming event. Those are fine goals to have, but you can't stop there, because they are not that motivating. "If you look at the data, the sustainability of those vanity-based goals is unreliable—we tend to peter out on our efforts once we start reaching a little bit of the goal," Kristin Kirkpatrick, registered dietitian, author, and manager of Wellness Nutrition Services at the Cleveland Clinic Wellness Institute, told me. I can relate—I can't tell you how many times I've cleaned up my diet, started feeling more energized, and then told myself some version of "I'm so healthy I can eat whatever I want, and it won't have any negative effects," and backslid into some old, bad food choices that make me feel sluggish and puffy again. (I blame all those media stories about models and actresses who can "eat whatever they want" and still be camera ready—which my cognitive mind knows can't be true, but my ego wishes applied to me.)

You may have a goal of wanting to lose weight, which is completely understandable, particularly because we have a culture that has long prioritized thinness as a goal. But resist the urge to name weight loss as your primary motivator. "Everybody wants to eat to lose weight," Dr. Kopecky said. "Instead, I say please eat to be healthy, and if you eat healthy, your weight is really not that big of a deal."

How can weight not be that big of a deal? Our understanding of health has evolved. "It's not about weight or even body mass index (BMI). It's about your abdominal girth," Dr. Kopecky explained to me. "Your waist size is an indicator of your health because abdominal fat puts out pro-inflammatory chemicals that actually cause us to have artery disease, more cancers, and more Alzheimer's."

When I asked Dr. Steinbaum about it, she explained that the presence of belly fat indicates that there's an inability to process sugars effectively, which typically results in elevated glucose levels, blood pressure, and triglycerides, while HDL, which is the good cholesterol, tends to be low. This confluence of symptoms—known as metabolic syndrome—is associated with diabetes, metabolic dysfunction-associated steatotic liver disease (MASLD), neurological disorders, polycystic ovarian syndrome, cancer, and cardiovascular disease.

So if you want to set a body-related goal, make it about reducing your waist size, and not about the number on the scale. According to an analysis of data collected in the Women's Health Initiative Study that was published in the premier journal *JAMA,* a waist size under thirty-five inches significantly lowers your risk of all-cause mortality as well as death from cardiovascular disease and cancer.[2]

Let's take a step back and look at the etymology of the word *diet,* which we closely associate with losing weight. The word is of Greek origin, from the word *diaita,* which means "a way of life." A way of life is very different from losing weight. It means you're practicing or even embracing a lifestyle, not trying to lose something.

It's better to make a health- and longevity-related goal. For example, Kirkpatrick shared with me that her motivation for eating healthy has far more to do with maximizing her brainspan: "I don't want my brain to start declining rapidly at sixty-five, and I develop dementia while my body is hanging on until I'm eighty," she confessed. That vision is what helps her keep her carb content moderate and avoid sugar. Excessive carbs and sugar have such a clear connection to dementia that certain forms of dementia are nicknamed "type 3 diabetes." "If you restructure your goals towards longevity, you're much more likely to stick to them," Kirkpatrick explains.

I agree with her. Ask yourself what healthspan-, brainspan-, and lifespan-related goals you have. Are you seeking to reverse a condition such as type 2 diabetes, chronic kidney disease, or something autoimmune-related, such as rheumatoid arthritis or irritable bowel syndrome? Do you want to improve your numbers, such as blood pressure, glucose, triglycerides, or bone density? Do you want to reduce or delay the risk of something that runs in your family, such as cardiovascular disease or dementia? Or do you want to live with health and vitality to ninety, a hundred, and beyond? Be honest with yourself about your hopes and fears—they can be great motivators for making changes that last.

Once you have your why down, you're better equipped to make changes that support ageless aging.

WHAT TO EAT: THE AMAZING BENEFITS
OF ANTI-INFLAMMATORY FOOD

Plenty of diets are popular today, including keto, paleo, DASH, MIND, and MEND, to name just a few. It can be utterly confusing and even overwhelming. While there can be benefits to these approaches, Kirkpatrick told me the problem with many of these diets—particularly keto and paleo—is that they are too hard to sustain over the long term. Dr. Dean Ornish, founder of the Preventive Medicine Research Institute, puts it very simply, "In general, diets don't work. You really just want to stick to eating whole foods."

However, the one eating pattern that has continued to be held up as great for longevity, as well as improving healthspan and brainspan, is the Mediterranean diet. It isn't a prescription; it's a description of how people who tend to live for a long time with a low incidence of cardiovascular disease and who live around the Mediterranean region (one of the Blue Zones) tend to eat. It's been proven by the test of time as well as by scientific research, and it is the basis of the ageless aging approach to eating. (It also closely aligns with Valter Longo's longevity diet.)

Hallmarks of the Mediterranean diet include:

- Eat plenty of fruits, vegetables, whole grains, nuts, seeds, herbs, and spices every day—the more colorful, the better (for reasons I'll dive into shortly).
- Most of your animal protein should come from fish and seafood— at least two times per week—with poultry and dairy occasionally.
- Consume lots of extra-virgin olive oil, replacing other fats like butter and vegetable oils. Be sure to choose extra-virgin.
- Lean red meats can be eaten once in a while, but avoid processed meats, such as bacon and sausage.

- Avoid sugar.
- A little bit of red wine each day (for women, that means one 5-ounce glass) is okay, with plenty of water. The addition of green tea has also been found to be helpful—regular consumption is associated with a decrease in waist circumference and an improvement in metabolic syndrome.[3]

A major reason the Mediterranean diet is considered to be particularly healthy is that it's primarily anti-inflammatory. Inflammation is a response of the immune system, which is helpful when you have an injury that needs healing, or a virus or bacterium that needs warding off, but can be downright harmful when there is no invader to attack. The body can misidentify some foods as harmful and trigger an inflammatory response that never really goes away. This can contribute to pain, autoimmunity, and lowered immunity—especially when you continue eating that food. Importantly, inflammation is associated with nearly all diseases and chronic conditions, including those that women suffer from disproportionately, such as arthritis, autoimmune diseases, and even dementia. I would emphasize that as we get older, inflammation becomes a growing problem for most of us. Truly, to increase our healthspan to better match our lifespan, we need to keep inflammation tamped down, especially as we live longer.

In my personal experience, to enjoy noticeable anti-inflammatory effects (such as a reduction in joint pain), it helps to eliminate gluten and dairy as well, although the medical world has not reached consensus that these foods are inflammatory. The good news is there are many foods that have anti-inflammatory properties, such as:

- Fruits, vegetables, whole grains
- Walnuts, almonds, and other nuts
- Extra-virgin olive oil
- Turmeric, garlic, cinnamon, ginger, cayenne, and black pepper
- Red wine

In a nutshell, your goal should be to eat fewer ultra-processed, inflammatory foods and more of the whole, anti-inflammatory foods.

YOUR NUMBER-ONE PRIORITY: EAT THE RAINBOW

Instead of thinking about how many servings of fruits and vegetables you're going to have in a day, focus on seeking to eat lots of colors. Kirkpatrick advises eating five colors every day. "We shut down when we hear recommendations to eat seven fruits and vegetables a day, but if you focus on eating colors instead, it becomes a lot more doable, even fun," she says. Once you get used to it, you'll find that it's pretty easy. Stir-fries; salads loaded with chopped veggies, herbs, and beans (my husband and I call them "power salads"); soups with beans, greens, squashes and/or peppers; even a crudité platter with your favorite dip—these are all delicious ways to eat a rainbow at one sitting.

Why are colorful foods so good for you? Polyphenols are the phytonutrients in plants that give them their rich colors. They are also packed with nutritional benefits. About eight thousand different polyphenols have been identified. Some have achieved rock star status thanks to copious amounts of research that have established their benefits—such as resveratrol, the component in grape skins that gives red wine much of its health-promoting properties, and epigallocatechin gallate (EGCG), which lends green tea its health-boosting powers. There are thousands of others, and researchers are only beginning to unpack their power.

Most polyphenols have antioxidant properties, meaning they help reduce inflammation and protect us from environmental stressors such as sun damage and pollution. Many have also been tied to favorably influencing epigenetics, helping good genes stay turned on and bad genes turned off.

Of course, polyphenols aren't the only beneficial compounds in whole foods. There are vitamins, minerals, and fiber. Vitamins and minerals feed your cells, while fiber fills you up, helps bulk up your stool so that you eliminate more of the things your body doesn't need, and also feeds your beneficial gut bugs, who then go on to further digest your food and use it to manufacture neurotransmitters, fatty acids, and some vitamins.

While each of these components is important, it's the interplay between them that we are only beginning to understand. "We may never fully grasp all the nuances of how the components of whole foods influence physiology, because the complexity of nature's wisdom truly is mind-boggling," Dr. Kara Fitzgerald wrote in her book *Younger You*. All you have to do to reap the benefits of this awe-inspiring gift from nature is to start putting more colorful foods onto your plate and into your mouth.

Here are lists of colorful foods to try:

- **Red.** *Fruit:* cranberries, red apples, guava, pink grapefruit, pomegranate, raspberries, strawberries, tomatoes, watermelon. *Vegetables:* peppers, radishes. *Beans:* kidney beans, red lentils. *Herbs:* cayenne pepper, paprika. *Tea:* passionfruit.
- **Orange.** *Fruit:* apricots, cantaloupe, clementines, oranges, peaches, tangerines. *Vegetables:* acorn squash, butternut squash, carrots, pumpkin, sweet potato.
- **Yellow.** *Fruit:* bananas, grapefruit, lemons, mango, pineapple. *Vegetables:* delicata squash, spaghetti squash, summer squash, yellow peppers. *Grains:* corn, quinoa. *Beans:* chickpeas. *Herbs:* curry powder, ginger, turmeric. *Tea:* chamomile.
- **Green.** *Fruit:* avocado, green grapes, kiwi, papaya (when unripe). *Vegetables:* artichokes, asparagus, bok choy, broccoli, Brussels sprouts, cabbage, collard greens, green onions, kale, leeks, lettuce, scallions, spinach, tatsoi, watercress, zucchini. *Tea:* green, holy basil (also known as tulsi), mint. *Herbs:* basil, cilantro, dill, mint, oregano, parsley, rosemary, sage, thyme.
- **Purple.** *Fruit:* blackberries, blueberries, elderberries, grapes, plums, prunes. *Vegetables:* eggplant, purple cabbage, radicchio, red onions. *Herbs:* lavender.
- **Brown.** *Beans:* lentils. *Vegetables:* mushrooms *Sweets:* cacao, dark chocolate. *Beverages:* black tea, coffee.

- **White.** *Vegetables:* cauliflower, daikon radish, endive, parsnips, radishes, jicama. *Herbs:* garlic.
- **Black.** *Beans:* black beans. *Grains:* black rice, wild rice.

Easy Ways to Eat More Vegetables (Organic Whenever Possible)

1. **Pre-prep them.** You reach for the foods you can see, so keep some cut vegetables ready to go at eye level in glass containers in your refrigerator (you can buy them pre-cut—although they typically cost more than whole vegetables). Carrots, celery, broccoli florets, cauliflower florets, jicama sticks, and sliced fennel are all great snacks. Also, keep dips on hand to dip your crudité in: hummus, guacamole, a vinaigrette made with extra-virgin olive oil, and babaganoush all make snacking on raw veggies delicious.

2. **Add them to everything.** Load up your salads, eggs, wraps, and sandwiches with organic veggies. I love a simple green salad or your basic scrambled egg, but they also present the perfect opportunity to throw in more color with vegetables and fresh herbs. Spinach, peppers, and onions go great with scrambled eggs; a green salad with shredded carrots, chopped cucumbers, sliced black olives, and a little minced green or purple onion is even better. Layer thin matchsticks of radishes, purple cabbage, and carrots onto a wrap or sandwich.

3. **Swap out traditional rice and pasta for the veggie version.** Minced cauliflower makes a great alternative to rice (look for it in the frozen section—it's typically less expensive than a head of cauliflower, even organic, and only needs to be cooked in a pan with a little water or broth and salt). And all kinds of spiralized vegetables—zucchini, sweet potato, beets, and more—make a nutrient-dense substitute for noodles. You can find these pre-cut in the refrigerator case of the produce section, and sometimes in the freezer section, or invest in a spiralizer and make them yourself.

4. **Ferment them.** Multiple cultures around the world rely on fermented vegetables as a staple of their diet—sauerkraut in Eastern Europe, kimchi in Korea, soy sauce from China, and traditional cucumber pickles, which were mentioned in the Bible. You can ferment all kinds of vegetables or buy them already fermented, as many grocery stores are carrying an ever-wider array of fermented vegetable options. These are naturally probiotic and really great for your digestion and immunity.

5. **Add them to smoothies and soups.** Greens—especially the milder versions such as spinach and kale—make great additions to smoothies. They can be added frozen or fresh. And you can make a delicious soup out of nearly any vegetable (some of my favorites are broccoli, cauliflower, and sweet potato) by sautéing some onions and garlic, adding your favorite herbs and a little salt, then several handfuls of your vegetable, diced, and enough chicken or vegetable broth to cover. Add a tiny bit of coconut milk if you want it creamy (or skip if you don't), simmer until the veggies are tender, then blend with an immersion blender.

6. **Grate them.** Grated vegetables—broccoli stems, green cabbage, purple cabbage, carrots, Brussels sprouts—make a great crunchy slaw-like salad, and you'll get multiple servings of vegetables in one sitting.

7. **Air-fry them.** Sweet potato, jicama, and butternut squash all make great fries. Simply cut them into fry shapes, toss them in a tiny bit of extra-virgin olive oil and salt, and roast them in a traditional oven or put them in an air fryer for more crunch.

Colorful foods are typically complex carbohydrates, one of the three main categories of nutrients known as macronutrients. The other two are proteins and fats. Here's more information about each of the macronutrient categories, with guidance on what foods from each macronutrient category to swap in, and which to swap out.

Carbs

With the keto diet craze—and the Atkins diet before that—carbs have gotten a bad rap. But carbohydrates are an important part of the human diet. "Historically, we have been eating about 55 to 60 percent of our calories as carbs, *but* (and this is a big but) they're not the processed kind—they grow on a tree or a vine or come out of the ground," Kopecky told me.

Simply put, there are healthy carbs and less-healthy carbs. Healthy carbs are known as complex carbs—these are the colorful vegetables, fruits, and whole grains that come out of the ground with plenty of phytonutrients and fiber, which slows digestion and prevents a big blood sugar spike. By seeking to eat the rainbow you will be eating plenty of complex carbs, and that's a good thing. It's the less-healthy carbs—known as simple carbs, such as white bread, white rice, and pasta, which are refined and stripped of their fiber—that we want to minimize.

Eating a lot of refined carbs kicks off a negative spiral that can trap you in a cycle of craving more refined carbs and put you on the path to metabolic syndrome, an increased waist circumference, and a higher incidence of chronic disease.

That doesn't mean you can never eat pasta again. You can either replace it with pasta made from beans, quinoa, or corn (which has more protein and fiber than traditional pasta, is gluten-free, and tastes pretty darn good) or eat a smaller amount of it accompanied by more high-fiber foods. When I interviewed Valter Longo, he said: "People are accustomed to eating a bowl of pasta or rice with a little bit of whatever on top; it should be the other way around. It should be a ton of beans and vegetables and a little bit of pasta and maybe a sprinkle of cheese," along with a few good glugs of extra-virgin olive oil. "After you make the switch, it actually tastes a lot better," Longo says. This is coming from a native Italian who is no stranger to pasta and who grew up in one of the Blue Zones.

Carbs to swap out: Processed foods including white bread, regular pasta, white rice, pretzels, pita chips, potato chips, regular crackers, white-flour tortillas, cereal, candy, cookies, ice cream.

Carbs to swap in: 100 percent whole wheat bread, sprouted wheat bread (like Ezekiel's) or nut and seed bread, low-carb bread (like the ones made by Carbonaut), almond-flour tortillas, chickpea-flour tortillas, rolled or steel-cut oats, popcorn popped in extra-virgin olive oil, dark chocolate, sweets made with high-fiber flour (such as almond or coconut flour) and natural sugars (such as honey, maple syrup, or coconut sugar).

Proteins

When most people think protein, they think meat. While red meat, which includes beef and pork, isn't inherently bad, it is high in saturated fat, which has been linked to high LDL cholesterol (the bad kind) and increased risk of heart attack and stroke. (Full-fat dairy has the same problem.) Unless the animals are pasture-raised, which accounts for only a fraction of meat consumed in the United States, the animals live miserable lives confined to feedlots. If you do indulge, I suggest organic, pasture-raised meat. The same with eggs.

A better choice for animal-based protein, and the one that centenarians eat the most, is fish and shellfish, particularly fatty fish such as salmon, sardines, anchovies, and herring, as they are rich in omega-3 fatty acids—an essential fat that our bodies need but can't make. (You should avoid fish that are bigger and higher on the food chain, such as tuna and swordfish, as they are more likely to be highly contaminated by mercury.)

Salmon is my favorite, and we eat it all the time. However, there is a lot of confusion about what kind to buy, wild or farmed. On the one hand, wild is lower in fat and calories than farmed and higher in omega-3 fatty acids, which reduce inflammation. However, farming of fish has improved dramatically, with more humane conditions for the fish and less environmental impact, while still delivering plenty of nutrition at a lower cost, typically, than wild. I often buy farmed salmon, but I buy it from a source I trust who vets the farms they buy from carefully. (Whole Foods is usually a great source for farmed fish.)

Some poultry is good, too—chicken, turkey, and eggs, all preferably pasture-raised and organic, both for the birds' sake and for yours, as the meat is richer in omega-3s when they can forage for their natural diet.

Plants can also provide a lot of protein, particularly beans and other legumes, nuts, and seeds. Even fruits and vegetables contain some protein. So by aiming to eat the rainbow, you will be getting a lot of it. We generally don't need all that much protein, about 0.33 grams of protein per pound of bodyweight, according to Valter Longo. That means 50 grams per day if you weigh 150 pounds. For reference, one egg contains 6 grams of protein, a four-ounce salmon filet has 23 grams, and a half cup of chickpeas has 20 grams.

However, to preserve our muscle mass, which tends to decline with age, we need to eat more protein once we get past age sixty-five. While Longo recommends that we make our primary source of protein legumes, after age sixty-five he suggests adding in more fish, eggs, and white meat poultry.

Proteins to swap in: Beans and other legumes (black beans, black-eyed peas, chickpeas, edamame, kidney beans, peas, pinto beans, white beans), nuts (almonds, cashews, pistachios, walnuts), seeds (pumpkin seeds, sunflower seeds, tahini—a paste of ground sesame seeds), small wild fatty fish (anchovies, cod, salmon, sardines), shellfish (clams, Gulf shrimp, mussels, oysters), chicken, turkey.

Proteins to swap out: Beef, pork, lamb, veal, bacon, hot dogs, salami, sausage.

Simple Ways to Eat Less Red Meat

Cut out processed meats. If you're eating red meat throughout the day, start by eliminating processed meats such as sausage, bacon, hot dogs, and deli meats. Eating less processed meat decreases your risk of cancer, heart disease, diabetes, dementia, and premature aging. One 2021 study found that eating a hot dog could take thirty-six minutes off your healthspan. At the same time, researchers concluded, "Substituting only ten percent of daily caloric intake from beef and processed meat for fruits, vegetables, nuts, legumes and selected seafood could offer substantial health improvements of 48 minutes [of healthy life] gained per person per day and a 33 percent reduction in dietary carbon footprint."[4]

Cut down on the number of servings and the size of the servings. If you're having red meat for lunch and dinner, reduce the portion size or just have it at one meal. When you do eat it, use the meat as more of a condiment than the star of the show (use one piece of roast beef on your sandwich and load up with fermented sauerkraut, or add some grated beets or sautéed mushrooms to the ground beef you use to make burgers so that you can use a smaller amount of beef). You don't need to wholly go without; rather, slowly retrain your palate and your habits to be happy with less red meat.

Swap in seafood or poultry. Turkey and salmon burgers are delicious, as are fish or shrimp tacos, chicken meatballs, and chicken or turkey chili. (My husband loves my turkey burgers with truffle salt and caramelized onions on a vegan bun.) Try a little smoked salmon on a chef's salad instead of ham, or in a wrap instead of roast beef.

Add in a meaty taste. "Umami" is a salty, savory, meaty taste that comes from foods such as soy sauce, miso, toasted nuts and seeds (and nut and seed butters), smoky spices such as cumin and smoked paprika, and mushrooms. Adding in this so-called fifth taste element (the other four are sweet, salty, sour, and bitter) can make the absence of or reduction in meat less noticeable.

Reach for plant-based alternatives. Lentils, chickpeas, and soybeans (whether whole, as in edamame, or in foods such as tofu or, my favorite, tempeh) can provide plenty of protein with none of the saturated fat of beef. The experts I interviewed all advised avoiding faux meats—such as the Impossible burger—because they are processed foods, high in fats. It's fine to have them once in a while, but you don't want to swap out a daily meat habit with a daily faux meat one.

Fats

There are definitely good fats, like extra-virgin olive oil and avocados, that have beneficial and anti-inflammatory properties. However, we're eating more harmful fats now than we did years ago—primarily vegetable oils that create inflammation, such as soybean oil, corn oil, safflower oil, sunflower oil, and canola oil. In addition, too much saturated fat from sources like red meat and full-fat dairy has been shown to lower lifespan and increase rates of cancer, heart attack, and death from all causes. On the flip side, healthy oils—like extra-virgin olive oil, avocado oil, and nut oils—have beneficial anti-inflammatory properties.

Fats to swap out: Bacon grease, lard, vegetable and seed oils (including in things like salad dressings and mayonnaise), fried foods.

Fats to swap in: Avocados, olives, ghee, extra-virgin olive oil, avocado oil, nut oils.

WHAT *NOT* TO EAT

As much as I believe in the power of adding healthy foods to your diet, you also have to stop eating—or dramatically lower your consumption of—the foods that are harmful to health. Especially those that contribute to inflammation.

Of the inflammatory foods, sugar is the absolute worst, for several reasons:

- When you eat sugar, which includes refined carbs such as bread, pasta, and white rice, your body breaks it down into glucose. In response, your body secretes insulin, which cues cells to let glucose in and get it out of the bloodstream. When you are eating refined carbs and sugars regularly, your insulin receptors get burned out and no longer receive the message to shuttle glucose into the cells. Thus, glucose levels *and* insulin levels stay high. High insulin cues the body to store fat and to crave more sugary foods. And persistently elevated blood sugar levels can lead to insulin resistance and increased risk of diabetes.

- When there is excess glucose on hand, it will bond with either a protein, a lipid (fat), or DNA through a process called glycation. Once glycated, that protein, lipid, or genetic material becomes brittle. This can happen in skin cells (so sugar makes you look older as well as age internally), brain cells, eye cells . . . everywhere in the body. Glycation is especially damaging to brain cells and explains why dementia is sometimes known as "type 3 diabetes." It's also the driving force behind many of the negative effects of diabetes, such as cataracts, neuropathy, and neurological problems. If you are prediabetic, have been diagnosed with metabolic syndrome, or are nervous about getting dementia, eliminating or dramatically reducing your sugar and refined carb consumption needs to be your top goal.

- It's almost impossible to eliminate sugar completely. It's in pretty much everything we eat, even fruits and veggies. It's refined sugar that we need to think of as toxic and remove from our diet. If you pick up any of the foods in your pantry and read the labels, you will likely see sugar listed in the ingredient list of almost all of them. And because the industry uses so many sneaky names for sugar in their ingredient list—I've seen lists of fifty or more such names, including brown rice syrup, dextrose, and turbinado—food manufacturers are now required to list "added sugars" in the nutrition panel. So always check how many grams of sugar there are in any food you're considering buying, paying special attention to the added sugars line, as these aren't the sugars that are naturally contained within that food, but are added to it in order to alter the taste and craveability of the food.

Tied with sugar at the top of the list of foods to avoid are ultra-processed foods—cookies, crackers, and packaged snacks, what Dr. Kopecky defines as "the things we all know we shouldn't eat, but of course we do." It's common sense to not eat foods that have been manufactured into something that in no way resembles its whole form, but it's not common practice. Dr. Kopecky told me, "Sixty percent of our calories now are from ultra-processed foods, which have a lot of bad things in them—inflammatory vegetable oils, sugars, and endocrine-disrupting compounds—that affect our metabolic health. So, we actually gain more weight by eating these."

Instead of grabbing that bag of chips, pop some popcorn in extra-virgin olive oil (popcorn is a whole grain, after all). Try roasted seaweed for a little salty crunch, or kale chips—which can be absolutely delicious with just a little extra-virgin olive oil, salt, and pepper! (Although a little grated Parmesan cheese on top is pretty tasty, too.) If you really want a bagged snack, try sweet potato chips cooked in avocado oil, or roasted beet chips.

Of course, I'm not expecting that you will never eat sweet and/or ultra-processed foods again. Just make them a rare treat. Get the junk food out of your pantry, so that you're not eating it every day. But if you go out and get ice cream once in a while, that's a pleasure you should enjoy. "There's a big difference between having a hot dog at the ballpark once or twice a summer and having one once or twice a week," Dr. Kirkpatrick said.

Or if you want to go out to eat with friends and they want pizza, go with them and enjoy. Choose a thin crust with veggie toppings for your pizza and have it with some salad, and that's a pretty healthy meal. Plus most places now have gluten-free options, which taste terrific.

Another big piece of the holistic recipe for increasing healthspan, brainspan, and lifespan is the social benefits of sharing a meal with friends and loved ones, enjoying conversation and community, and de-stressing. Ken and my major entertainment and social outing these days is going out to dinner or to dinner parties with friends, eating yummy food, and having a glass of wine. It creates the mood for relaxation, fun, and conversation—and frankly, my husband and I could both use more of those things. I don't want to take that away from anyone. Even Valter Longo agrees: "Some violations once in a while are actually healthy." I'll drink to that!

HOW MUCH TO EAT: LET YOUR
HUNGER BE YOUR GUIDE

It's not just what you eat, but how much you eat. Whatever you're eating, you want to be mindful of the quantity of food you're consuming. Kirkpatrick told me, "If you can just manage your hunger and fullness, that alone can help you make peace with food." How do you do that? She advises listening more closely to your body's cues.

Put simply: Don't wait until you get ravenous to eat. By the same token, don't eat until you are stuffed. "You would never go to the gas station and, once your tank is full, keep filling it so the gas spills out on your shoes. But we do that with our body every day," she told me. Aim for staying in a nice middle range between a little hungry and satisfied (which is different from full). This helps keep your hormones that regulate hunger—including insulin and leptin—in balance.

Like most things in life, there is a spectrum to hunger. This list, taken from the University of California, Berkeley, website, lays it out clearly. Basically, you want to keep your hunger between a 4 and a 7 on this scale.

Fullness to Hunger Spectrum

10 – Extremely stuffed, nauseous

9 – Stuffed, very uncomfortable

8 – Overfull, somewhat uncomfortable

7 – Full, but not uncomfortable

6 – Satisfied, but could eat more

5 – Starting to feel hungry

4 – Hungry, stomach growling

3 – Uncomfortably hungry, distracted, irritable

2 – Very hungry, low energy, weak, dizzy

1 – Starving, low energy, very weak

Source: University of California Berkeley, wellness-hungersatietyscale.pdf (berkeley.edu)

That means eating when you start to feel hungry, or when you are legitimately hungry and your stomach is growling, but not waiting so long that you're starving or low energy—because then your hormones will be screaming at you to get as many calories in your belly as you can as quickly as you can. By the same token, you want to stop eating when you are satisfied and comfortable—not when you couldn't eat another morsel and feel like you need to lie down and unbutton your pants.

"There should never be a moment during the day where you feel stuffed," Kirkpatrick says. That's because fullness is something we only feel after our insulin levels have risen in response to the rise in blood sugar that follows a meal, and after food has reached the small intestines, which then release chemical messengers that signal the body has enough sustenance for now—a process that takes about twenty minutes to kick in. If you're wolfing down your food, or not paying attention to what you're putting into your mouth, you can eat well past the point of satiety and end up feeling overly full. It may be difficult, if not impossible, to eat more slowly and/or stop eating before you are stuffed if you have food addictions or an eating disorder, or if you have been eating ultra-processed foods that are formulated to be addictive. In addition, many of us have received a lot of programming around cleaning our plates. There can be a lot to unwind, and the process may take some time. Simply raising your awareness of how full you feel as you're eating and after you've finished is a gentle and important place to start.

WHEN TO EAT: INTERMITTENT FASTING

One of the few things that longevity and health experts agree on pretty much across the board is that *when* you eat matters as much as *what* you eat. In his book *Lifespan*, Harvard professor and longevity expert David Sinclair writes that if you do only one thing to positively affect your longevity, it's "eat less often." This understanding emerged from the research on caloric restriction conducted on mice at the University of California at Los Angeles by Dr. Roy Walford. Caloric restriction is a dietary regimen that reduces food intake without incurring malnutrition—and according to Walford's research, eating less has been linked to increased longevity . . . if you're a mouse. Dr. Walford himself famously experimented with caloric restriction, limiting his own diet to 1,600 calories daily for the last thirty years of his life. Yet not even a strict diet could save Dr. Walford from amyotrophic lateral sclerosis (ALS), also known as Lou Gehrig's disease, which he suffered from for twelve years before dying at age seventy-nine. Although perhaps his regimen helped—the average life expectancy for someone with ALS is two to five years.

Dr. Volter Longo worked in Walford's lab and realized that it was nearly impossible to restrict calories without inciting malnutrition in humans. From this knowledge, he developed a practice you've likely heard of, and perhaps even engaged in—intermittent fasting, which, if done right, has real health and longevity benefits. If done incorrectly, it can actually cause health problems.

When done safely, intermittent fasting offers the following benefits:

- Helps you not overeat.
- Restores insulin sensitivity.
- Reduces inflammation more effectively than other diets.
- Helps reduce incidence of breast cancer, Alzheimer's disease, arthritis, asthma, multiple sclerosis, and stroke.[5]
- Improves sleep. Since you're not doing the work of digestion, you can rest more deeply.
- Boosts cellular repair. Fasting appears to trigger the cleanup process of removing waste material from cells and recycling damaged cells.
- Increases human growth hormone, which facilitates fat burning and muscle building.
- Improves gene expression. More helpful genes (like tumor-suppressor genes) are turned on, while bad genes (like pro-inflammatory genes) are turned off.

- Restores metabolic flexibility. When you go for longer periods without eating, your body will likely burn through any stored glucose and be coaxed into burning fat for fuel. "By hour eight, nine, ten, eleven, or twelve, you're starting to break down some fat," Longo says, which helps with weight loss, particularly when it's abdominal fat.
- Burns abdominal fat. A 2014 review found that study participants who practiced intermittent fasting lost between 4 and 7 percent of their waist circumference over a period of twenty-four weeks.[6]

Keep in mind that intermittent fasting is not really fasting at all, but what Dr. Longo describes as *time-restricted feeding*. And the sweet spot, according to Dr. Longo, is twelve to thirteen hours without food. Dr. Felice Gersh, board-certified in obstetrics and gynecology as well as in integrative medicine and a globally renowned expert in women's health and complex disease management, agrees: "It's really important that women have a fasting period overnight of twelve to thirteen hours." The benefits are enormous, including weight loss, better metabolic health, and improved cardiovascular health.

However, there are many biohackers and longevity gurus who advocate and practice longer windows of fasting, up to sixteen hours between meals, on a regular basis. Dr. Longo told me that this is not necessarily a healthy practice. A twelve- or thirteen-hour window means you eat breakfast and "breakfast is the most important meal of the day," Longo told me. "Skipping breakfast and doing a longer fast of fourteen or sixteen hours is consistently associated with shorter lifespan, more cardiovascular disease, hypoglycemia, and the formation of gallstones." In particular for women, as we age, we need more protein to help prevent osteoporosis, and it can be hard to eat enough protein in a smaller eating window.

Keeping the window between meals to twelve or thirteen hours is not that hard to do. For instance, I try to finish dinner by 8:30 p.m., and don't have anything to eat until the next morning at 8:30 a.m.

It has the added benefit of helping me sleep better. I do this on most days, which is what Dr. Longo suggests.

There are other forms of intermittent fasting—including the 5:2 approach, where you eat normally for five days and then fast or eat only about 500 calories or less for two days, and the alternate-day fast, where you eat normally one day and then either fast or eat only 500 calories the next. I recommend the daily 12/12 approach because it is so doable, but if there's a reason why one of these other approaches works better for you and your life, by all means give it a try.

No matter which approach you choose, every day you want to stop eating three hours before bedtime. Your body is designed to repair and restore itself during sleep—not digest food, which distracts it from the important restorative functions of sleep. When you stop eating three hours before bedtime, it impacts your sleep positively because your metabolism doesn't have to be working.

The one caveat is that you still need to eat healthily during your eating window. "Some people think, 'As long as I'm eating within a twelve-hour period, I can eat whatever I want.' That's not the case," Kirkpatrick says. Intermittent fasting isn't a replacement for healthy eating; it's a plus to healthy eating.

HYDRATION AND BEYOND FOR MAINTENANCE AND HEALING

Water is incredibly important to your health, as the human body consists of 60 percent water. A human can survive only a handful of days without water; you could survive up to two months without food.

Hydration helps with circulation, delivering nutrients to and flushing away waste products from all your cells. Water lubricates your joints, promotes cognitive function, regulates body temperature, and reduces headaches and body aches. It also appears to increase lifespan as well as healthspan. A 2023 study found that people ages fifty-five to sixty-six with serum sodium levels—a marker of dehydration—on the higher end of normal (above 142 millimoles per liter) had a 50 percent higher risk of having a biological age that was higher than their chronological age, and that was associated with a higher risk of chronic disease and premature mortality.[7]

Clearly, if we want to age agelessly, we've got to drink up. The rule of thumb is to drink half of your body weight in ounces of water each day—although herbal tea also counts toward your hydration goals. (Regular coffee and tea, although healthy beverages, contain caffeine, which is dehydrating.) That means if you're 150 pounds, you need 75 ounces, or about 9½ eight-ounce glasses of water. It helps to either make a note of every glass you drink in your daily planner, or buy a big water bottle that holds as many ounces as you need each day and pour your glasses out of it. (Or both.) Eating water-rich foods, such as fruits and vegetables, also helps meet your hydration needs, both because those foods contain water and because they are likely to replace dehydrating, high-sodium processed foods (think cookies, crackers, and chips). I start every morning with a cup of warm water with the juice of about one-quarter of a lemon, which helps jump-start my hydration and my digestion, and delivers a little bit of vitamin C.

Because of contaminants in the water supply, it helps to filter your tap water (to remove lead from old pipes, chlorine, and other toxins) or drink spring water. Basic carbon filters (like a Brita) work well, as long as you change them frequently—otherwise they can start leaching the things they've filtered out back into the water.

Beyond water, what beverages are healthspan-, brainspan-, and lifespan-positive? Coffee and tea are antioxidant-rich beverages with documented health benefits. Coffee is helpful for regulating gene expression and protecting liver health, while tea, particularly green tea, is widely hailed as an overall health booster. Try to find a brand of tea that is organic. When it comes to coffee, it, too, should be organic and shade grown (so it doesn't contribute to deforestation) and/or Fair Trade (so that the people who grow and pick the beans are paid a living wage). And while a little almond, oat, or regular milk or unsweetened coconut creamer is fine, you want to wean yourself off sweetening your hot morning beverage with sugar. A little sprinkle of stevia or monkfruit goes a long way; a bit of honey is okay, too.

You can also make yourself what I call a mega-beverage—a golden milk made with turmeric (look for a pre-blended, unsweetened powder at Whole Foods), a matcha latte, or a cacao drink. Turmeric, matcha, and cacao are all superfoods, but you don't have to eat them; you can drink them. I make my mega-beverage by heating a little almond or oat milk, sweetening it with a little stevia, and then whisking a tablespoon or two of the milk with a few teaspoons of the powder in the bottom of my mug so that it's well blended before pouring in the rest of the heated milk. Delicious, and a perfect late morning or midafternoon pick-me-up.

When it comes to alcohol consumption, more and more evidence suggests that "it fundamentally affects DNA," according to Dr. Tim Naimi, director of the University of Victoria's Canadian Institute for Substance Use Research. However, the exact effects vary depending on the type and amount of alcohol consumed. In general, one 5-ounce glass of wine per day for women may actually have health benefits, such as reducing stress and the risk of developing some types of cardiovascular disease, but it can impact our sleep negatively. (You can see how the different ingredients of our holistic recipe influence each other.) Red wine *is* a part of the Mediterranean diet, after all, in moderate amounts.

Nearly all the experts I spoke with said they enjoyed a glass of wine with dinner (even a couple who officially espouse avoiding it altogether, but I'm not naming names). To be clear, a glass of wine means one 5-ounce glass, not two or three glasses. Personally, I seek out organic or biodynamic wines to minimize pesticides. There are so many excellent wineries that are moving in this direction. If you prefer spirits, avoid sugary mixers and have them on the rocks or with seltzer and a squeeze of lemon or lime. One serving of spirits is one ounce. Indulge, but don't overindulge.

YOUR GUT MICROBIOME

We've been hearing a lot more about the importance of the gut microbiome and how it plays an essential role in digestion and even our overall health. Let's try to unpack this a little bit more.

The gut microbiome is a complex population of bacteria, viruses, and fungi that live in your digestive system, influencing areas of health such as digestion, immunity, heart health, and even mental health. When the gut microbiome is out of balance, your body might not be able to absorb nutrients effectively, and it may cause inflammation. A diversity of gut microbes is beneficial to our health, which means eating a wide variety of nutrient-dense foods such as fruits, vegetables, legumes, nuts, and seeds. That's the diet we've been talking about. In addition, eating adequate amounts of fiber can help encourage the growth of healthy bacteria and promote regularity. Prebiotics and probiotics, such as fermented foods like kombucha, sauerkraut, and kimchi, enhance the diversity of gut microbes and decrease molecular signs of inflammation, according to researchers at the Stanford School of Medicine.

Taking a prebiotic and/or a probiotic supplement can also be a valuable tool. I find a probiotic with a big diversity of bacteria works well for me. Researchers are currently looking into how changes in the gut microbiome can affect metabolic health, disease risk, and even preventive care.

HACKING YOUR HEALTH AND LONGEVITY WITH OCCASIONAL LONGER PERIODS OF FASTING

Intermittent fasting is time-restricted eating, like the twelve-to-thirteen-hour window discussed earlier in this chapter. On the other hand, fasting is not eating and drinking water only (or water and herbal tea only) for a longer period of time, one to five days. "Short periods of fasting or a fasting-mimicking diet can have beneficial effects that last long after the fasting period is through," Dr. Longo told me. A fasting-mimicking diet is designed to give you the benefits of fasting while still consuming a small amount of food. Typically lasting five days, a fast-mimicking diet is very low in calories and contains carefully calculated macronutrients to provide the nutrients your body needs without blocking the beneficial responses that are triggered by fasting. In addition to being much easier than water-only fasting, fast-mimicking has been shown to reduce body weight, fat stores, blood pressure, triglycerides, total cholesterol, and low-density lipoprotein cholesterol (the so-called bad kind), fasting glucose levels, and C-reactive protein (a marker of inflammation).[8]

The foods that Dr. Longo espouses eating on your fast-mimicking days come straight from the Blue Zones and are recognized as super-ingredients for longevity. They include non-starchy vegetables such as greens and cauliflower, plant-based proteins such as beans and tofu, healthy fats such as olive oil and avocado, nuts, and seeds. What I find most amazing—and I've tried his ProLon five-day fasting-mimicking diet kit—is that while the food is minimal, it helps curb your appetite, so you don't feel too hungry.

More is definitely not better when it comes to fasting. Dr. Longo reminded me, "Once you get to a certain period, the body actually enters a thrifty mode and then it slows down the metabolism, so it does not run out of stored energy." You want to avoid getting into the thrifty mode. He suggests following a fasting-mimicking plan for five days at a time, three or four times a year, as an overall insurance policy for better health.

FOOD AS MEDICINE

There are times in everyone's life when we are dodging an illness or even facing a serious disease or condition. And these times are when food becomes more than just sustenance; it becomes medicine.

Dean Ornish explains, "I was trained, like all doctors, to view heart disease, diabetes, breast cancer, and even Alzheimer's disease as being fundamentally different diseases with different diagnoses and treatments. They're really the same disease manifesting in different forms. They all share the same underlying biological mechanisms such as chronic inflammation, oxidative stress, telomere shortening, and angiogenesis. Each of these mechanisms is influenced by what we eat." He absolutely believes that food can be a highly effective way to fight disease. "There's a difference between how you eat on an everyday basis versus how you eat to conquer disease When you're using food as medicine, that's when you tighten the reins and stick to a narrower range of foods," Ornish told me.

While our understanding of how our diets directly influence our risk of developing and odds of treating disease is continuing to evolve, here is a quick guide to the eating plans that have been developed and implemented to treat specific conditions.

Diet	Hallmarks of diet	Diseases and conditions that it benefits
Ketogenic diet	Keep carb consumption low (about 50 grams or less per day, generally) while upping intake of healthy fats and non-starchy vegetables so that the body burns fat for fuel (instead of glucose, which is derived from carbs).	Epilepsy,[9] cancer,[10] dementia[11]
DASH (Dietary Approaches to Stop Hypertension) diet	Eat foods that are rich in potassium, calcium, and magnesium (minerals that help control blood pressure—found in fruits, vegetables, nuts, and seeds) and reduce consumption of sodium, saturated fat (from red meat, processed meats, and full-fat dairy), and sugar (five servings of sugary foods and drinks or less per week).	High blood pressure[12]

Diet	Hallmarks of diet	Diseases and conditions that it benefits
MIND (Mediterranean-Intervention for Neurodegenerative Delay) DASH diet	Eat more of these ten foods: green, leafy vegetables; all other vegetables; berries; nuts; olive oil; whole grains; fish; beans; poultry; wine (no more than one glass per day). And minimize these five foods: butter and margarine; cheese; red meat; fried food; pastries and sweets.	Dementia (reduces risk)[13]
Low-FODMAP (fermentable oligosaccharides, disaccharides, monosaccharides, and polyols) diet	This is an elimination diet that takes out all foods that contain FODMAPs, types of short-chain carbohydrates that can trigger digestive distress after eating in some people. Then you reintroduce them one by one to determine which you do or do not tolerate. High-FODMAP foods to eliminate include: dairy-based milk, yogurt, and ice cream; wheat; beans; artichokes; asparagus; onions; garlic; apples; cherries; pears; and peaches.	Irritable bowel syndrome (IBS) and small intestinal bacterial overgrowth (SIBO)[14]

Diet	Hallmarks of diet	Diseases and conditions that it benefits
AIP (autoimmune protocol) diet	Also an elimination diet that removes all potentially inflammatory foods for an initial period of thirty to ninety days, including grains, legumes, nuts, seeds, nightshade vegetables, dairy, alcohol, tobacco, coffee, oils, processed foods, and sugar. In their place, the protocol includes plenty of non-nightshade vegetables, fruit, minimally processed meat, fermented foods, and bone broth. After the initial period, eliminated foods are reintroduced one by one to determine which aren't tolerated and should be minimized over the long term.	Multiple sclerosis, rheumatoid arthritis, inflammatory bowel disease, Crohn's disease,[15] Hashimoto's disease
Gluten-free diet	This eating plan eliminates all sources of gluten, including wheat, bulgur, rye, malt, and barley. In addition to being found in most breads, pasta, cereal, and crackers, gluten can also hide in beer, soy sauce, sauces, stews, and soups (where flour is often used as a thickener).	Celiac disease,[16] autoimmune thyroid issues[17]

CUTTING-EDGE NUTRITIONAL DEVELOPMENTS

- **Precision nutrition.** Let's face it, we're all different. The rules of basic nutrition aside, there are so many individual factors that influence how your body uses food. These include your genetics, your microbiome, your lifestyle, your stress, your environment, and more. For all these reasons, the future of nutrition is in finding ways to personalize dietary recommendations to the individual. (This is true of all healthcare, not just nutrition, by the way, but more on that in Chapter 7.) Two techniques some providers are already using—as well as many individuals, as these tests are available to consumers, too—include:

  - **Nutrigenomics.** You likely know that you can get a DNA test to determine your ancestry and which diseases, conditions, and traits you are more predisposed to, but our ability to map the genome has also created a genetics test that can give you insight into which nutrients you may need more of and which foods may not agree with you. Known as nutrigenomics, this test, which uses a saliva sample, analyzes approximately seventy genes to look for specific variants that may be impacting how your body interacts with specific foods and nutrients. For example, the report will show you if you have a genetic predisposition to a lactose or gluten intolerance, how well you tend to metabolize certain components of food (such as saturated fat and caffeine), if you are prone to high triglyceride levels, and even if you have an elevated preference for sugar or fat. Knowing what your particular body needs more of—and doesn't tolerate well—can help you personalize your dietary plan. It can also be validating to learn that you're not making it up that your stomach feels upset after eating dairy because you have the genetic variant associated with lactose intolerance, for example. The sophistication of these tests—and our understanding of different genotypes—is continually evolving. Many different companies offer these tests; a search for "nutrigenomics test" will yield a lot of results. You can find one at the price point and level of service that works for you. Some offer only reports; others offer a consultation with a dietitian or nutritionist.

- ◦ **Microbiome testing.** We already discussed the importance of the gut microbiome for your digestive and overall health. Today scientists are exploring the ways in which the gut microbiome can be manipulated to improve health. Now you can submit a stool sample to get your microbiome analyzed for specific strains of bacteria. The results of these tests typically come with food and lifestyle recommendations to get your particular microbiome to a healthier place. Like nutrigenomics, the science of how impactful the results of a microbiome test can be is still inconclusive. I've done three microbiome tests, and each time the foods I was told to avoid and to prioritize were completely different. However, each time I took the test, I was at different levels of stress, general health, and digestive health. It made perfect sense to me. Still, as the science evolves, microbiome tests will become an even more important part of precision medicine. The leaders in the field at the time of this writing are the companies Viome and Floré, but the field is quickly evolving.

- **Continuous glucose monitors.** These wearable devices, which, as the name suggests, continuously monitor your glucose levels, are gaining enormous popularity. The benefit of such a device is that it helps you understand how your particular body reacts to specific foods by giving you hard numbers of how much your glucose levels rise after eating, exercising, and periods of stress and relaxation. It gives you great insight into what kinds of foods and lifestyle practices help you avoid blood sugar spikes that tank your energy and kick off a cascade of negative hormonal reactions. Say, for example, you've found a dark chocolate bar that claims to contain no sugar (because it's sweetened with a sugar alcohol, such as erythritol, that allegedly doesn't affect blood sugar levels), but when you eat it, your continuous glucose monitor shows that you do indeed see a significant rise in blood sugar. Or maybe that you don't! A typical glucose monitor requires a finger prick and test strips; a CGM attaches to the back of your arm or to your belly and can give continual readouts, either on an app on your phone or on a small device that you wear in your pocket. Traditionally, CGMs are prescribed by your doctor if you are prediabetic or have been diagnosed with diabetes, but that is changing. Some companies, including AgelessRX and Signos, offer them to consumers. CGMs typically require a subscription that costs about $150–$200 per month and may or may not come with access to a nutritionist and other support.

FOOD: WHERE TO BEGIN

If you do one thing: Cut out sugar as much as you possibly can
Functional medicine doctor Beth McDougall told me that eating sugar "is like kicking your immune system in the balls." Eliminating it will help lower your risk of a host of chronic diseases, improve your energy levels, and, over time, change your palate so you won't crave it as much.

If you're a total beginner: Add more colorful whole foods to every meal and eliminate ultra-processed foods
The colorful foods will crowd out the ultra-processed stuff, their fiber will fill you up, and their polyphenols will help keep your good genes turned on and your bad genes turned off. They'll also start changing your taste buds. Eliminating the ultra-processed foods will give you more energy and improve your health on a cellular level.

If you already eat a healthy diet regularly and are ready to take it to the next level: Incorporate intermittent fasting
Give yourself a twelve- or thirteen-hour break from eating each day, including the three hours before bedtime. Along the way, do as Dan Buettner, author of *The Blue Zone* series of books, suggests and

front-load your calorie intake to earlier in the day. If you're already doing intermittent fasting, make plans for your first five-day fast-mimicking diet. Dr. Longo's ProLon kit is pricey but makes it easier, eliminating your sense of hunger. There's even a pill that might be available by now—that's right, a pill—called Mimio that is in beta testing at this writing. It has gone through more than a hundred clinical trials and is described as the "world's first biometric supplement to mimic fasting on a molecular level."

AGELESS AGING HACKS
TO UNLEASH THE POWER OF FOOD

Save money and time while improving your health with organic frozen fruits and vegetables

Frozen produce may seem like an inferior option to fresh, but really, it's just the opposite. "When you flash-freeze something it retains the cellular integrity and the nutrients, so it's actually healthier than foods that were grown in another hemisphere and picked three weeks ago," Dr. Kopecky told me. Better yet, "frozen produce costs about a third or half as much, with more nutritive value." Frozen produce is also incredibly convenient. For example, adding frozen chopped spinach or kale to a pot of soup ups the nutrition and the taste without a lot of washing and chopping.

Buy extra local produce when in season and freeze it

You can make it an outing and pick your own berries or squash, and then you'll also be serving up some memories each time you pull those strawberries out of the freezer.

If money is an issue, spring for organic only for the Dirty Dozen

The pesticides on conventionally grown produce can wreak havoc on your health, but organic produce can be harder to find and more expensive. "Eating organic can certainly help reduce cancers," says Dr. Kopecky. But you don't have to buy everything organic. Kopecky advises staying up to date on what's on the yearly Dirty Dozen list of the most contaminated types of produce, created and maintained by the Environmental Working Group (www.ewg.org/foodnews/dirty -dozen.php), and prioritizing buying those types of produce in their organic forms. As I write this, the Dirty Dozen (in alphabetical order) are: apples, blueberries, cherries, grapes, green beans, greens (kale, mustard, and collards), nectarines, peaches, pears, peppers (bell peppers and hot peppers), spinach, and strawberries.

Drink silica-rich water

Christopher Exley, PhD, professor of bioinorganic chemistry at Keele University in the United Kingdom, studies Alzheimer's and has observed high levels of aluminum in the brains of people who suffered from the disease. In his research, Exley has determined that silica binds with aluminum and can help escort it out of the body. There are twelve bottled waters identified by waterpurificationguide.com that naturally contain high levels of silica, including Fiji Natural Artesian Water, Gerolsteiner Sparkling Natural Mineral Water, and Volvic Natural Spring Water. However, all bottled waters have a big environmental footprint, which is the downside.

Stick to extra-virgin olive oil

Not all olive oils are created equal. According to the PREDIMED study, study participants who followed the Mediterranean diet with an extra daily supplement of either extra-virgin olive oil or nuts experienced a 30 percent reduction in risk of cardiovascular events compared to a control group that was only told to eat a low-fat diet.[18] Because extra-virgin olive oil is cold-pressed (not extracted using chemicals or heat the way standard olive oil often is), the thirty different types of polyphenols contained in the peppery green oil that reduce inflammation and target the hallmarks of aging are preserved. Extra-virgin olive oil is also lower in acidity, tastes better, and works great whether you drizzle it over a salad or cook with it (using medium to low heat so as to preserve its beneficial properties).

Sip organic bone broth

Organic bone broth is a superfood containing a wide variety of vitamins, minerals, and amino acids that nourish your tissues and provide essential nutrients for healthy body functioning. It is especially high in calcium and magnesium, which are important for building bones, regulating hormones, and detoxifying the body. Since it is a rich source of L-glutamine, an amino acid that helps to heal the lining of the gut and improves digestion, bone broth is also great for gut health. It also contains prebiotics, which are beneficial bacteria in the gut that help to reduce inflammation, improve nutrient absorption, and promote better digestion and gut health.

There's more. Bone broth is believed to help reduce joint pain, promote joint healing, and improve mobility due to its high content of collagen, which is necessary for healthy cartilage and joint construction. You can buy it prepackaged in many grocery stores now (in the broth aisle), or you can make your own in a stockpot on your stove (letting the bones and any aromatic veggies you want to include, such as carrots, onion, and celery, simmer in plenty of water for eight to twelve hours) or in an Instant Pot (which only takes three to four hours). There are hundreds of great recipes online. If you are vegetarian, a vegetable broth that includes nutrient-rich wakame seaweed and mushrooms is a great alternative—Google "vegetarian bone broth" for a wide array of recipe options. And sprinkle nutritional yeast on top for a boost in B vitamins and a great cheesy taste.

6

$\bullet$

THE MAGIC OF SLEEP

Sleep can be elusive, especially for women, especially as we grow older. Not only is getting enough sleep challenging, but the very subject of sleep can feel incredibly stressful. We know sleep is vital to our health (and I'll break down all the ways it influences your healthspan and your brainspan in just a bit), but it doesn't always feel like it's something in our control. It's also easy to obsess over—I often do—and then you lose sleep over losing sleep

A confession: sleep is definitely *not* my superpower. I often struggle with it. For me, it's not falling asleep, which I do easily, but staying asleep. I wake up pretty regularly at 2 or 3 a.m., and then it's a crapshoot as to whether I will fall back asleep on my own, go back to sleep with the aid of a supplement or prescription med, or just toss and turn the rest of the night. The good news is that as I've been doing research and talking to the experts on sleep for this book, I've been experimenting, trying out the suggestions I'm learning about, and my sleep has dramatically improved. So, there's hope. If I can do it, so can you!

I know I'm not alone in the struggle for a good night's rest. A full third of the adult population experiences chronic insomnia, according to a study by the National Library of Medicine.[1] The challenge of sleep seems to be greater for women than men. Anecdotally, in an informal

Age Wave poll, women said the number-one daily health and fitness issue they are concerned with is their lack of sleep. As we enter and move through perimenopause, menopause, and postmenopause, sleep can become a nightmare, as the lack of estrogen and progesterone—and the resulting hot flashes, night sweats, increased irritability, and impaired ability to relax—can have a negative effect on both falling asleep and staying asleep.

No matter what is impeding you from getting the sleep your body needs, it can be remedied. Dr. Aric Prather, a psychologist and sleep expert at the University of California, San Francisco, who treats insomnia and is the author of the book *The Sleep Prescription*, told me, "There's no instance where I, as a sleep doctor, have to throw up my hands and say, 'Your sleep is broken. I'm sorry. There's nothing we can do.' Sleep is something that's built into our DNA—it's just that we need to remove the barriers that get in the way of allowing it to happen naturally."

In addition, there are lots of new solutions in our toolbox thanks to the increased availability of relatively affordable and easy-to-use apps that apply guided meditation and breathing exercises as well as cognitive behavioral therapy techniques to sleeplessness. This means we don't have to rely on habit-forming medications or grogginess-inducing supplements to get the sleep our bodies and minds so desperately need. Even if you have a truly disruptive sleep disorder, such as sleep apnea, there are many treatments available now that can get you back on the path to restful sleep.

We're also seeing an exciting shift that recognizes sleep as part of a bigger discipline—circadian rhythm medicine—which has deepened our understanding of how our internal clock regulates our sleep cycles. It's given us even more and better tools to improve our sleep. I would emphasize that this is a new science with evolving insights and knowledge that will continue to shed light on how we can improve our sleep.

So, we're not doomed to lie awake for hours each night, stressing about how tired we're going to be the next day. Let's unpack all of this, starting with why sleep matters so much in the first place.

THE BENEFITS OF SLEEP

Sleep is a master regulator of our health—a vital sign as important to our ageless aging as fitness and nutrition. Our understanding of the *why* is still evolving. "We used to believe sleep was the time that the body rests, but when you look at the brain during certain sleep cycles, you see it is very, very active," explains Dr. Gavin Britz, director of the Houston Methodist Neurological Institute and the Candy and Tom Knudson Centennial Chair of Neurosurgery. "It's clear that something essential happens during sleep."

It's only been since 2013 that we've understood a major reason that sleep is so vital for brain health. That's the year when Dr. Maiken Nedergaard and her colleagues at the University of Rochester Medical Center discovered the glymphatic system—a series of channels within the brain that use cerebrospinal fluid to flush away metabolic waste products during deep sleep. It's a kind of detox. Additionally, while we're sleeping the brain is in a calmer state requiring less energy, which means our metabolism slows and we produce fewer toxic waste products. Not only do we take out the trash while we sleep, we simultaneously accumulate less trash in the first place.

Beyond the brain, sleep helps us repair tissue throughout the body, balance hormone levels, nourish our epigenome so that good genes stay turned on and bad genes stay turned off, and even consolidate our memories.

There's more. Other benefits of sleep include:

- **Positively impacts your appetite and metabolism.** Sleep helps regulate hormones, such as ghrelin and leptin, that influence how hungry you feel.
- **Improves cognitive function and emotional regulation.** Sleep enhances your ability to learn, store memories, make decisions, and navigate emotional and social challenges with relative composure. That helps you relate better to other people and boosts positive feelings toward others.

- **Boosts overall health.** Physiologically, sleep has a slew of benefits, including strengthening our immune system and helping us to maintain a healthy cardiovascular system. It also reduces the risk of certain diseases such as depression and diabetes.
- **Promotes more ageless aging.** From a holistic perspective, sleep helps you have more energy for exercise—and exercising helps you sleep more soundly. A good night's sleep also gives you energy to pursue activities that are meaningful to you and helps you tap into your sense of purpose. And, as we all know, when you're sleeping well, you look better.

Dr. Phyllis Zee, director of the Center for Circadian and Sleep Medicine at the Feinberg School of Medicine, Northwestern University, Chicago, summed it up perfectly for me: "It turns out when you give people their sleep back, so many things improve. Their mood, their relationships, their other behavioral choices all improve. It's such a powerful tool."

Assess Your Sleep Quality

This simple, five-question survey is known as the SATED questionnaire—an acronym that stands for satisfaction with sleep, alertness during waking hours, timing of sleep, sleep efficiency, and sleep duration. It was developed by sleep researchers as a simple way for individuals to get an objective look at the quality of their sleep. While it isn't scientific per se (there are no studies that link certain scores to certain health outcomes), it does help you see your own sleep patterns more clearly and can give you a good "before" and "after" snapshot to gauge the effectiveness of any sleep interventions you try.

To use it, answer the questions and add up your score. A score of 0 indicates poor sleep health, and a score of 10 indicates great sleep health.

	Rarely/never (0 points)	Sometimes (1 point)	Always (2 points)
Satisfaction. Are you satisfied with your sleep?			
Alertness. Do you stay awake all day without dozing?			
Timing. Are you asleep (or trying to sleep) between 2 a.m. and 4 a.m.?			
Efficiency. Do you spend less than thirty minutes awake at night? (This includes the time it takes to fall asleep and the awakenings from sleep.)			
Duration. Do you sleep between six and eight hours per day?			

If you're reading this list and thinking, "My poor sleep is going to take me down," remember—sleep is a habit and, just as it can be lost, it can be regained. It may be out of whack, but it can get better. Also, you don't need to stress about occasional nights of bad sleep or short-lived rough patches. "Even with all the best strategies in place, you can still have a bad night's sleep, and that's okay," Zee said. "It's about how you manage your sleep on average, because the negative health effects are more closely tied to chronic sleep deprivation or chronically short habitual sleep."

Before we get into sleep hygiene and strategies to improve your sleep, it's helpful to understand more about sleep itself—how much you need, the different stages of sleep, and how you can address sleep issues by taking better care of your internal clock.

WHEN IT COMES TO SLEEP, IT'S NOT JUST QUANTITY, IT'S QUALITY

Just a decade ago, celebrities like Kim Kardashian and Martha Stewart would brag about how little sleep they got. (Kim Kardashian: five hours nightly. Martha Stewart: four hours nightly.) We used to think that less is more: five or six hours of sleep was all you needed to perform at top levels and take on the world. We now know this is not true. While some people are genetically wired in such a way that they truly only require four to five hours of sleep to function well—they are known as familial natural short sleepers—the genetic mutation is extremely rare. "Most people who think they're natural short sleepers are not," Dr. Prather told me. "And there is fairly clear evidence that very short sleep—five hours or less—is really bad for you."

It's hard to pinpoint the exact amount of sleep we should aim for. We have individual needs that evolve as we age, and little science to guide us because sleep recommendations are generally based on small studies of people between the ages of eighteen and sixty-four.

Prather told me that the national societies devoted to sleep, such as the American Academy of Sleep Medicine and the Sleep Research Society, all suggest that up until age sixty-four, we should aim for at least seven hours per night to maintain optimal health. For those of us sixty-five and older (myself included), the data just isn't there to make broad recommendations. "My guess is in the next decade we will have more information to make that kind of recommendation," Dr. Prather said. "What we know now is that as people get into the sixth and seventh decades of life, they usually get less sleep."

Like most things related to health, there are differences between the sexes. "Men have more sleep apnea and other sleep issues across all age groups. However, once women hit menopause, they catch up on sleep problems—insomnia, poor-quality sleep, sleep apnea, and short sleep duration—rapidly," Dr. Zee told me. She admits that we don't know if sleeping less, and less well, as we age is a natural progression because we require less sleep, or if it's a symptom and co-factor of physiological decline. She does say that women's sleep issues later in life are likely related to their higher incidence of autoimmune conditions compared to men, and that estrogen and progesterone are protective against sleep apnea. So when those hormones decline, our proclivity to sleep apnea rises.

It's not just duration of sleep that matters; it's also quality. As you may remember if you have children, in those newborn days when your sleep was regularly interrupted, all you longed for was a solid stretch of at least a few hours. That's because consecutive hours of sleep enable your body to go through a more complete sleep cycle and experience each of the four different stages of sleep, each serving a different function. When you are regularly awakened, you can get trapped in a light sleep cycle, which won't let your body perform all the important functions that happen throughout the various sleep cycles, leaving you feeling more tired.

When I asked Dr. Zee if you're better off sleeping four straight hours of uninterrupted sleep or seven hours of somebody elbowing you all night long, she confessed, "I don't know the answer to that, but I would probably choose the four hours of uninterrupted sleep."

A better metric than number of hours spent in bed is how much sleep it takes for you to wake up feeling well rested.

The Four Stages of Sleep

In a typical night, you'll go through somewhere between four and six 90-minute sleep cycles. Each part of the cycle plays an important role.

Stage 1: N1. This shortest phase of light sleep lasts just one to ten minutes, when you are falling asleep. Technically, you do come to semi-consciousness at the end of each sleep cycle and return to N1 sleep, but you don't spend much time here before heading into stage 2.

Stage 2: N2. During this phase your body temperature drops, your breathing and heart rate slow, and your muscles relax. Throughout the night, you spend about half your time in this stage of sleep.

Stage 3: N3. This is deep sleep, or slow-wave sleep, when your brain waves are moving their slowest, which is important for memory consolidation and washing away toxic waste products from the brain via the glymphatic system. It's also believed to play a role in immunity. In fact, when people have been deprived of deep sleep in a research setting, their risk factors for disease go up. During this phase, your blood pressure and metabolic rate dip.

Stage 4: REM. When your eyes are moving behind your lids, you're in REM (rapid eye movement) sleep, which is important for mood regulation and emotional memory processing. It's also linked to learning and creativity, which makes sense, as this is the stage of sleep when the most vivid dreams occur. We tend to spend less time in REM sleep as we age.

THE NEWISH SCIENCE OF CIRCADIAN RHYTHMS

As I mentioned earlier, sleep is actually a subset of circadian rhythm medicine. Circadian rhythms refer to the physical, mental, and behavioral changes that occur in the body roughly every twenty-four hours in response to light and darkness. Your circadian rhythms control not only the sleep/wake cycle, but also the release of hormones such as cortisol and melatonin, fluctuations in body temperature and metabolism, your sense of hunger, gene expression, a whole host of cellular processes, and nearly every other body function. Circadian rhythms are influenced by your diet, exercise, and environmental cues. They're also very personal to each of us.

What we do know for sure is that understanding circadian rhythms gives us another set of tools for nurturing our sleep. The most potent tool in this new toolbox is light. Dr. Steven Lockley, associate professor of medicine at Harvard and one of the world's top experts on circadian rhythms and sleep, puts it this way: "The absolute key to healthy sleep and circadian rhythms is stable, regularly timed daily light and dark exposure. Given that most of our body systems express circadian rhythms, ensuring proper alignment of our internal circadian clocks, starting with the management of light, will have major impacts on human health."

That's not quite as easy as it sounds. "Most of us are totally out of sync with our biological clock, because we live by the clock on the wall, which often doesn't jibe with our internal clock," Zee explained. The wall clock is the same every day (except for the days we spring forward or fall back), while our internal clock changes with the sun. When your daily activities get out of sync with your circadian rhythms— as is often the case, especially for shift workers—there's an increased risk for heart disease, metabolic disorders, and cognitive disorders. For example, science has found that jet lag disrupts the microbiome in both mice and humans.[2] Even sleeping in on the weekends—known as "social jet lag"—can cause negative changes in your microbiome, and has been linked to drinking more sugar-sweetened beverages and eating fewer fruits and vegetables.[3]

Unsurprisingly, your circadian rhythm plays a huge role in how well you sleep. This internal clock is personal to you and influenced by your underlying physiological preference for a daily sleep/wake cycle that's part of your genetic makeup. Dr. Zee explained that the most powerful way to get your circadian rhythm into a better cycle is to get savvier about your exposure to light, especially morning light.

Morning daylight is more in the blue end of the light spectrum, which is stimulating, whereas the light at sunset, as well as candlelight and firelight, are farther into the red end of the light spectrum, which is calming. Even if you're blind or have low vision, your eyes will pick up signals from light and use them to regulate your circadian clock. Even when it's cloudy outside that morning light still counts, as it is about five times brighter than your typical indoor lightbulb. Dimming bright lights and exposing yourself to red light and even darkness at night is also important.

Light affects more than just sleep. Science has shown that the amount of light you get is associated with depression—think of seasonal affective disorder, the fancy term for the winter blues, which happen during the darkest times of the year.

SLEEP PRESSURE MATTERS, TOO

Besides circadian rhythms, the other biological mechanism that guides our sleep is sleep pressure, your body's innate drive to sleep that accumulates throughout the day. Sleep pressure is triggered by the buildup of a molecule in your brain known as adenosine, a byproduct of the process of creating and burning the molecule of energy known as adenosine triphosphate (ATP), the form of energy that fuels cellular processes throughout the body. In fact, caffeine wards off sleepiness by temporarily blocking the adenosine receptors in the brain. But that doesn't make adenosine go away—it still builds up, so when the caffeine wears off and the adenosine receptors are functional again, your built-up tiredness can feel almost overpowering.

Because sleep pressure can vary so much day to day and person to person, having a consistent bedtime isn't necessarily the answer (something I unpack more in the "Sleep Myths to Ignore" section of this chapter). For example, if you work a particularly long day at your desk and don't move much, then wind down by watching a thriller at night, you're probably not going to be tired at your usual bedtime. It's best to feel sleepy to start your bedtime routine and get into bed.

SETTING YOUR CIRCADIAN CLOCKS: YOUR DAYTIME TO-DO LIST TO SLEEP BETTER AT NIGHT

It's natural to think that a better night's sleep starts with your bed-time routine, but that's a fallacy. It actually starts as soon as you wake up. Arianna Huffington, the successful serial entrepreneur and author of *The Sleep Revolution*, told me, "The way I start my day is hugely important in determining what follows. And a big part of my morning ritual is about what I don't do. When I wake up, I don't start the day by looking at my smartphone. Instead, once I'm awake, I take a minute to breathe deeply, take in the sunlight, be grateful, and set my intention for the day." She's on to something, as her morning routine jibes with the following simple but powerful interventions sleep experts agree on. If you try them and don't conk out for seven solid hours of blissful sleep tonight, don't write them off. "The biggest shift that people have to make in trying to fix their insomnia is that it's never just about tonight," Dr. Prather told me. "It's about improving your sleep on average by working with your circadian rhythms."

- **Wake up at the same time every morning.** The most important thing you can do to normalize your sleep is to have a consistent wake-up schedule—even on days when you go to bed late, don't sleep well, or don't have to get up to go to work. Dr. Zee's rule is not to wake up more than one hour after your typical wake-up time during the week, and no more than two hours on your days off. Her mantra is: "Maintain the robustness of the rhythm."
- **Drink in that morning light.** Throw open your shades, or better yet, drink your morning cup of coffee outside or go for a short walk. Know that you're setting your circadian rhythm to help you be more alert during the day and sleepier at night. Even if it's cloudy, raining, or snowing, you'll still be getting energizing

blue light. Dr. Beth McDougall told me, "When the sun is rising, I go outside barefoot on the ground, watch the sunrise, and do some stretching outside."

- **Get plenty of movement.** If I don't move enough, I don't sleep enough. Remember from Chapter 4 that daily movement has many benefits, including better sleep quality.

- **Set aside time during the day to worry.** One reason we have trouble falling back to sleep if we awaken during the night is that the wheels start turning—and not in a good way. "No one ever says, 'I was awake in the middle of the night, and I was only thinking of good things,'" Dr. Prather said. He suggests setting aside some time during your day to write down what you're anxious about. Doing this brain dump is a cognitive behavioral therapy technique that can protect your peace of mind in the middle of the night.

- **Choose a caffeine cutoff time.** Caffeine has a half-life of four to six hours, so you want to have your last cup of coffee by either noon or 2 p.m. This is somewhat individual, but ideally no caffeine within eight hours of bedtime.

- **Dim lights around sundown.** Turn off bright overhead lights. Instead, light candles, watch the sunset, stare at the fire.

- **Close the kitchen.** Have your last bite to eat at least three hours before bedtime, so your body doesn't have to devote precious sleep time to digestion.

- **Develop a sleep ritual.** "The more consistent you keep those things like putting on your pajamas, watching TV on the couch, and turning down the lights, the more you create a stronger conditioned response," Dr. Prather told me, so that when you get in bed, "it's like a hammer coming down."

Arianna Huffington shared her nighttime sleep ritual: a warm bath with Epsom salts (which contain magnesium that can help you relax) and a candle flickering nearby. "Sometimes I have a cup of chamomile or lavender tea if I want something warm and comforting before going to bed. And I have a specific time at night when I regularly turn off my devices—and gently escort them out of my bedroom."

- **Dress for sleep.** Huffington told me, "I don't sleep in my workout clothes, as I used to (think of the mixed messages that sends to the brain!), but make sure to wear pajamas or T-shirts that are dedicated to sleep." If you run hot at night, wear as little as possible.

- **Adjust the temperature.** Sleep researchers like the University of California at San Francisco's Ying-Hui Fu, PhD, and Louis Ptacek, MD, suggest something as simple as keeping your room temperature at 65°F to help improve sleep duration and morning alertness. This is something I do, and it really seems to help. That's because your core body temperature naturally drops during sleep—if your room, bed, or pajamas are too warm, it will be harder to fall and stay asleep. You can even buy cooling mattress toppers if you tend to feel too hot at night.

Treatable Sleep Interferences

There are many things beyond garden-variety stress and anxiety-related insomnia that can prevent you from getting good sleep. If you consistently wake up feeling tired in the morning, no matter how many hours you spent in bed, these might be impacting you. They are all treatable.

Sleep apnea. More severe than simple snoring, sleep apnea occurs when your airways close while you're sleeping, essentially blocking off the flow of oxygen and choking you to the point that you wake up, at least five times per hour and as often as every minute, to gasp for air. Aside from causing sleepiness, headaches, and sore throat the next day, sleep apnea also takes a big toll on cardiovascular and cognitive health. The good news is that sleep apnea can be remedied either with airway pressure devices (such as a CPAP machine) or oral devices that can restore regularity to your airflow. And as you'll read in the hacks section of this chapter, you can now evaluate yourself for sleep apnea using a home test, rather than having to wait for an appointment to spend the night in a sleep lab.

Menopause—sort of. The changing hormones of perimenopause and menopause can interfere with restful sleep in a few different ways. Hot flashes and changes in body temperature can make you feel like you're too hot to sleep, for example. But, Dr. Zee cautions, "Don't chalk your sleep problems up to hormones and think there's nothing you can do about it. There are lifestyle factors that can be modified. There are also mood disorders that become more prominent during that period, such as depression, which can interfere with your sleep."

Restless leg syndrome. This is characterized by an unpleasant feeling in the legs when the body is at rest—so strong that you feel an almost uncontrollable urge to move the legs. It's twice as common in women as in men, and menopause increases the likelihood and severity of symptoms. Restless leg syndrome can be the result of an iron deficiency; it's also typically associated with not getting enough movement during the day. If twitchy legs are keeping you up at night, schedule an appointment with your physician.

Depression. Depression has a tight bond to sleep—people who experience chronic insomnia have a ten-times-higher risk of developing depression than people who sleep well, and 75 percent of people with depression experience insomnia. Because the two are so intertwined, you don't want to treat only your insomnia or your depression; you want to focus on both to minimize the risk of backsliding. There's some early evidence that cognitive behavioral therapy for insomnia can help improve sleep in people with depression, and increases the chance of a lessening of depressive symptoms, according to Johns Hopkins Medicine.[4]

SLEEP MYTHS TO IGNORE

Sometimes the thing that's most detrimental to our quality of sleep is misinformation. Here are some of the most pervasive myths that keep us from getting good sleep.

Myth #1: You must have a consistent bedtime

Yes, having a bedtime routine is helpful as it cues your body to get ready for sleep. But tying that routine to a specific time isn't always helpful, because depending on what happened during the day, you may not be sleepy yet, and getting into bed before you're tired can be anxiety-inducing. Conversely, you may have had to get up early that morning, or had a physically busy day, which has caused your sleep pressure to build up earlier than usual, and waiting until a set time to get into bed can mean you miss your sleep window.

If you tend to wake up in the middle of the night, or wake up too early, Dr. Prather told me that pushing your bedtime back later, even for just a few nights, can help snap your sleep back in place. Even though you may get less sleep overall, you'll get more consecutive hours of sleep and, thus, more completed sleep cycles and a greater feeling of restfulness.

Myth #2: A "good night's sleep" does not include any waking up in the middle of the night

It is perfectly natural to wake up during the night, perhaps because you have to go to the bathroom, or because you hear a noise, or simply because you've completed a sleep cycle and you have a few moments of wakefulness (which you may not even remember) before starting again with light sleep.

Don't let the very fact that you're awake in the middle of the night be a source of stress. Remind yourself that it's natural—and then follow the tips in the "What to Do When You Wake Up in the Middle of the Night" section of this chapter.

Myth #3: No screentime whatsoever before bed

Yes, blue light is stimulating and, mostly, the light emitted from screens is blue. But there are many apps and even settings built into your device's operating system to tone down the blue light once the sun goes down. Plus, watching a show or reading on your Kindle can be a nurturing and relaxing part of your bedtime routine. Prather tells me the trick is to make sure the content isn't stimulating—stick with something soothing like *The Great British Baking Show* instead of something gripping, like a murder mystery. For this same reason, it's best to avoid emailing, texting, or scrolling through social media or your news feeds just before bedtime.

WHAT TO DO WHEN YOU WAKE UP
IN THE MIDDLE OF THE NIGHT

According to Dr. Prather, "Lying awake in bed perpetuates insomnia by stoking your anxiety and weakening your mind's association that bed means sleep." This is a main tenet of cognitive behavioral therapy for insomnia, the gold standard for sleep intervention. Dr. Prather recommends giving yourself twenty minutes, tops, to try to drift off, but if you're still awake after that point, "you've got to get out of bed until you feel sleepy again." When you do, avoid things that are mentally stimulating and stick to quieter pursuits, such as knitting, meditating, coloring, or reading a boring book—or listen to a guided meditation, sleep story, or sleep-inducing podcast (you'll be surprised by how many results you get when you search for one). Keep the lights dim, and don't worry that getting up will only make you more awake. Dr. Prather says, "Your drive to sleep continues to build sleepiness, even when you're awake."

If you really, really don't want to get out of bed, or can't for whatever reason, change your position by sitting up or even lying down the opposite way so your head is where your feet normally go. Once you feel sleepy again, you can resume your normal lying-down position.

Dr. Prather tells me that middle-of-the-night wakefulness is simply a pattern that needs rewiring, both by changing your physical location and by chipping away at the catastrophizing that typically happens when we find ourselves awake at 3 a.m. *again.* "As people get older, they wake up more. Period. It's not something to be worried about and worrying about it is only making the problem worse," he says.

Thanks to what I discovered in researching this chapter, I've been embracing a consistent wakeup time of 6 a.m. and making sure to expose myself to natural light as soon as I'm up. (We are fortunate to have a view to the east, so I've been soaking in the sunrise.) Before I go to sleep, and if I wake up in the middle of the night, I've been using the app Breathwrk to guide me through a sleep-inducing breathing exercise. While I do still wake up in the wee hours, I try not to start thinking—I immediately turn on the app and fill my head with the breathing exercise. It has definitely been helping. My daughter-in-law also gifted me a product called Vagus Nerve Pillow Mist, which contains a blend of essential oils, including lavender, lime, and rosemary, purported to stimulate the vagus nerve. It smells great, and when I feel really anxious I use it sparingly. However, if I use it routinely, I feel brain fog in the morning. As a side note, research suggests that stimulating the vagus nerve—the primary nerve of your parasympathetic nervous system, which winds from your brainstem through your neck, heart, and lungs and down to your gut and is a key player in digestion, immunity, and regulating your heart rate—can be useful as a remedy for insomnia.[5] One other way to activate the vagus nerve is cold exposure, especially on your neck. Try an ice pack or ice-cold washcloth on your neck for a few minutes before sleep. I'll go into more detail about the vagus nerve and stress in Chapter 9.

Something else that has helped is to put a moratorium on talking about work with my husband after dinner (not easy to do, because we work together). Those conversations can get my wheels turning when they should be slowing down as my sleep pressure rises. Instead, I've been reading or watching predictable rom-coms—and no offense to romance fans, but they put me right to sleep! I've made measurable progress, and the relief that brings improves my sleep even more.

To Nap or Not to Nap?

I asked Dr. Prather about naps, and he said short naps of ten to thirty minutes can be mentally and physically refreshing and part of a healthy sleep routine, but research confirms that longer naps tend to leave you feeling sleepier.[6] If you're napping because you're so tired you can't keep your eyes open, it's a sign you need more sleep at night. Rather than sleeping during the day, which can reduce your sleep pressure and interrupt your circadian rhythm, Prather suggests going to bed earlier so you can catch up on some of that lost sleep without throwing your master cycle out of whack.

THE DOS AND DON'TS OF SLEEP MEDS AND SUPPLEMENTS

- **Melatonin** is not technically a sleep aid. Rather, it's a cue to your circadian rhythm that the time for sleep is near—it signals darkness to your brain. The experts I spoke to said melatonin was helpful for resetting your master clock if your circadian rhythm has gotten out of whack, as is the case in jet lag. But they suggested using a very small amount, like 1 to 3 mg—not the 5 or even 10 mg that are in the typical drugstore melatonin supplements that people pop at bedtime, which typically makes you feel groggy even eight hours after you take it. If you want to stimulate your own internal melatonin production, be vigilant about dimming your lights at night, because exposure to bright light after dark can shut off the production of melatonin.

- **Benzodiazepine sleep medications,** such as Valium (diazepam), Xanax (alprazolam), Ativan (lorazepam), and Klonopin (clonazepam), work by binding to GABA receptors in the brain, which produces feelings of relaxation and sleepiness. The issue with these meds is that they are addictive, meaning it can become hard to fall asleep without them, which then creates anxiety around sleeping without them. They also mask the true problem of what's causing your insomnia, Prather says. "They're good for acute stress, but with chronic use, you may be eroding the brain health that you're trying to save by getting more sleep." It's important to note that benzodiazepines, as well as the drugs I cover in the next entry on this list, are emphasized on the American Geriatrics Society's Beers Criteria® list of potentially inappropriate drugs for older adults and discouraged as first-line therapy for insomnia, because they have risks associated with falls, delirium, and other cognitive effects that may impact concentration and brain function.

- **Zolpidem, Ambien, and other sleep medications.** These can offer short-term relief from insomnia or sleeplessness, but you can build up tolerance quickly and they can be addicting. They also come with potential side effects such as increased fall risk, drowsiness, confusion, memory problems, and impaired thinking and balance. Sleepwalking or sleep-driving have also been reported, with people not remembering they even did these things.

CUTTING-EDGE SLEEP DEVELOPMENTS

- **Personalized, digitized cognitive behavioral therapy for sleep.** This is the gold standard for improving sleep. Until recently, cognitive behavioral therapy for insomnia was available only through sleep labs, which are often expensive and have long waiting lists. However, multiple apps now offer access to a personalized set of tools and recommendations based on CBT-I, including Somryst (which has approval from the Food and Drug Administration [FDA]; somryst.com), the Sleep Reset (which also gives you access to a real live sleep coach; thesleepreset.com), and Sleepio (which may be covered by your insurance; sleepio.com). These apps guide you through cognitive exercises, relaxation techniques, and meditations geared toward your unique sleep challenges, and each has gone through clinical trials that demonstrate their effectiveness.

- **Somnox sleep robot.** This may sound high-tech, but it is actually an avocado-shaped pillow that you can cradle while lying in bed (somnox.com). The sleep robot expands and contracts to help you subconsciously match your breathing to its rhythms, helping you naturally enter a calmer, more sleep-receptive space. It also can play guided meditations or lead you through specific breathing exercises that you can choose through its companion app.

- **Light therapy sleep masks** use orange light at night to stimulate the production of melatonin and then gentle blue light in the morning to wake you up. They may even incorporate speakers to play relaxing music or guided meditations. Aside from benefiting everyday sleep, these masks can also be programmed to help you recover from jet lag or the sleep disruptions associated with shift work. Available from Lumos (lumos.tech) and Dreamlight (dreamlight.tech).

- **Dynamic circadian lighting.** Dr. Zee tells me that soon we'll have access to indoor lighting that automatically changes the ratio of blue to red light emitted from the bulbs to more closely mimic the way natural light changes throughout the day and night. There are already a small number of such lamps on the market, including the SkyView Wellness Table from BIOS Lighting (bioslighting.com), which cycles through four different lighting modes, designed to emulate sunrise, daylight, sunset, and nighttime.

- **Glymphatic system–stimulating cap.** A team of neuroscience researchers and engineers at Houston Methodist, Rice University, and Baylor College of Medicine are developing a "sleeping cap" to analyze and stimulate the activity of the glymphatic system in the hopes that even people who sleep poorly can rid their brains of waste products efficiently. The idea is that this cap will be portable and easy to use, so that essential workers, such as deployed soldiers, can protect their neurocognitive health even when their sleep is challenged.

- **Electrotherapy stimulation handheld device.** Bono Sleep (bonowellness.com) is a small device that fits in the palm of your hand and emits electrical pulses that you can feel (and control the intensity of), which the company claims calms your nervous system. You can also choose to heat the device in order to warm your hand—warmth in your extremities has been shown to dilate blood vessels and, paradoxically, encourage heat loss that helps bring down your core temperature, cuing the body to sleep.[7]
- **At-home sleep apnea tests.** The Lofta WatchPAT test is an FDA-approved portable breathing monitor that can assess whether you have sleep apnea by measuring blood oxygen levels, peripheral arterial tone, heart rate, physical activity (how much you toss and turn), snoring, and chest motion. It involves a night spent sleeping in your own bed wearing one monitor on your finger, another on your wrist, and another on your chest with cords that connect the devices. The WatchPAT sends your results to a sleep doctor for evaluation, and you get the results in one to two weeks—no appointments or night spent in the sleep lab needed. You need a prescription to get the test, so you'll want to check in with your primary care physician or sleep specialist, who can determine whether this is a good fit for assessing your sleep quality.

SLEEP: WHERE TO BEGIN

If you do just one thing: Devote time in bed to either sleep
or sex—nothing else

If you're awake and having difficulty falling asleep or staying asleep, and it's been twenty minutes, take a cue from cognitive behavioral therapy and either delay your bedtime until you feel truly tired, get out of bed, or at least switch positions.

If you're a total beginner: Nourish your circadian rhythms in the morning

Try keeping your wake-up time consistent and expose yourself to bright light first thing in the morning. "It helps train your circadian rhythms to be more in sync," which will benefit your sleep, advises Dr. Zee.

If you're already taking steps to improve your sleep but want to take it to the next level: Do a "worry brain dump" during the daytime

If you're like me and wake up in the middle of the night and your mind starts racing through your list of worries or your to-do list, take some time to write down your concerns and to-dos during the day. It's a cognitive behavorial therapy trick, the gold standard for solving sleep problems, that seems to alleviate middle-of-the-night anxiety. Remember Dr. Prather's words: "No one ever says, 'I was awake in the middle of the night, and I was only thinking of good things.'"

AGELESS AGING HACKS TO IMPROVE SLEEP

Have sex/an orgasm

Hopefully you've figured this out by now, but having an orgasm either by yourself or with a partner can help you drift off. Why? Having an orgasm releases several biochemical messengers that are thought to promote sleep, including oxytocin (which reduces the stress hormone cortisol), serotonin (which the body uses to make melatonin), and prolactin (which has been shown in a small 2021 pilot study to induce REM sleep).[8]

Use mouth tape

Breathing through your nose—with its built-in filtration and temperature-regulating systems—is better for you than breathing through your mouth. Nose breathing also stimulates the production of nitric oxide, which promotes vascular health. A social media trend that was popularized by author James Nestor in his book *Breath: The New Science of a Lost Art*, is using a small piece of skin-friendly tape to keep your mouth closed—and your breathing happening through your nose—while you sleep to prevent mouth breathing and snoring. Word of caution: If you have sleep apnea and tape your mouth shut, you could impede your ability to breathe. Only ever tape just the middle of your lips with a small piece of tape that is easy to remove, such as medical tape available at drugstores. You want to prevent your mouth from opening, not completely seal off your entire mouth.

Try non-sleep deep rest (NSDR)/yoga nidra

Yoga nidra is an age-old guided relaxation that talks you through systematically checking in with and then inviting every part of your body to relax. According to yogis, it is more restorative than a nap. Non-sleep deep rest (NSDR) is very similar to yoga nidra in that it also aims to get you into a deeply relaxed state that is not necessarily sleep. There are countless YouTube videos for both yoga nidra and NSDR. If you haven't tried it before, you're in for a treat—prepare to feel like a noodle.

Change your lightbulbs

At the very least, turn on your brightest lights and throw open your curtains and shades in the morning, then start to dim them around the time the sun goes down so that by the time it's dark outside, you don't have more light than you truly need to be able to see what you're doing. You could take it one step further and have certain lights or lamps with blue lights that are for daytime and then other lights or lamps with red lightbulbs for nighttime. Some LED bulbs can change the tone of their light through an adjustment of a dimmer or dial.

Breathe to induce sleep

Huffington told me, "Breathing is a favorite 'sleep hack' of mine. Counting out a few slow breaths is one of the techniques I use when

I'm having trouble falling sleep." She uses the 4-7-8 method, where you inhale quietly through the nose for four counts, hold your breath for seven counts, and then exhale through the mouth for eight counts. Breathwork gives your mind something to focus on, so you don't get stimulated by your internal chitchat. It also encourages you to breathe more deeply and engage your diaphragm, which helps to cue your body's relaxation response.

7

YOU ARE THE CEO OF YOUR OWN HEALTHCARE

It's a simple truth that taking better care of your health means taking better advantage of the healthcare system. That's not easy to do, but I'll walk you through it.

The healthcare system can be confusing, difficult to navigate, and not at all user-friendly. It's often siloed by whatever healthcare system you belong to and, within that system, further broken up by subspecialties. In addition, the system focuses almost exclusively on sick care, not wellness care or preventive care; if you're trying to increase your healthspan, brainspan, and lifespan, this can be frustrating.

On top of all that, the healthcare system wasn't really built for us women. Let's use pharmaceutical product testing as an example. It wasn't until 1986 that women were allowed—yes, allowed—to participate in clinical research and trials. And it wasn't until 2016 that the FDA issued guidance on clinical trial enrollments to include an equal number of women and men when possible. As a result, many pharmaceutical products haven't even been tested on women, making us more vulnerable to adverse effects from medications.

I hate to tell you there is more to consider with healthcare as a woman over fifty, but there is. When it comes to our health, less than half of all accredited medical schools in the United States require a geriatrics rotation. And the number of board-certified geriatricians in the United States fell by approximately 25 percent between 2000 and 2022.[1]

The takeaway? Like it or not, as we live longer, we women need to take charge of our own healthcare. This can be a tall order, but I will try to show you how to make the most of your healthcare experience.

It starts with a basic understanding of what you need to know and do and what's available to help you in this process. I'll also point to what's available if you want to look deeper into your health to be sure you're taking steps to increase your healthspan, brainspan, and possibly even your lifespan. By no means is this going to cover everything, but I hope it will help you have a clearer picture of how to take charge of your interactions with our nation's convoluted healthcare system.

THE HEALTHCARE PARADIGM SHIFT

Our parents and grandparents often put doctors up on pedestals and dutifully followed their orders. Today we have to be the CEO of our own healthcare. This doesn't mean you have to have all the answers or know the medical minutiae, but it does mean being more proactive and, wherever possible, taking more self-responsibility. It means your doctors are your partners and advisors—they can guide, conduct and interpret diagnostic tests, and make recommendations, but you have the primary seat at the decision table. Your advisory committee might also include your pharmacist, fitness instructor, chiropractor, acupuncturist, nutritionist, massage therapist, and a host of other alternative practitioners who help you manage your wellness. It's not self-indulgent to have a team of people helping you feel your best, as health is the most valuable asset you have.

SIX STEPS TO BUILDING A HEALTHIER
RELATIONSHIP WITH HEALTHCARE

So how do you become the CEO of your own health and create a healthier, less frustrating experience with the healthcare system? Here are six steps to help you get started.

1. **Find a primary care physician you trust and can relate to.**
   Every expert I talked to stressed how important it is to have a primary care doctor. Dr. Suzanne LeBlang, a Florida neuroradiologist, co-chief medical officer of the Focused Ultrasound Foundation, and the medical director for the Fibroid Education Center, told me, "You act as the CEO of your own healthcare by choosing the right doctor for you."

   This can admittedly be a difficult task, with many physician practices closed to new patients. Ask your friends, family, and colleagues to refer you to their favorite clinicians. Research your potential doctor's training, learn about their specialties, and read their reviews; you ideally want someone who is trained in preventive care and chronic disease management.

   A primary care physician is important because they are the one who will know everything that's going on with you and can help make your care more cohesive. Dr. Christina Pham, an internal medicine physician at UCSF Medical Center who has also been my doctor, told me, "Every time something happens that affects your health, even if it doesn't seem important, tell your primary care doctor. That way, there are two places where all your healthcare information resides—in your mind and in your physician's mind." You can't advocate for your health if you don't know your weight, blood pressure, cholesterol, blood sugar, and heart risk—this is what your annual checkups will tell you. Don't blow them off.

2. **Prepare for your doctor's visits in advance.** Many systems allot merely fifteen minutes per in-person visit—not enough time

for an in-depth conversation or to address multiple concerns. To help maximize these appointments, create a to-do list beforehand. Consider sending your questions in advance to optimize your doctor's time. You can do this through your

Other Healthcare Providers You May Want on Your Healthcare Team

Physicians

Functional medicine doctors

Integrative medicine doctors

Osteopaths

Naturopaths

Complementary care providers

Chiropractor

Acupuncturist

Herbalist

Homeopath

Massage therapist

Reiki master

Fitness trainer

Yoga/meditation teacher

Nutrition advisors

Nutritionist/dietitian

Health coach

Wellness coach

doctor's online portal, or by calling the office in advance and asking to leave a message for the doctor with their physician's assistant or nurse.

3. **Ask questions and advocate for yourself.** Bring up your concerns and ask pointed questions to help you understand whatever health situation you may be facing so you're able to make the best decisions. Dr. Pham shared, "In my relationships with my patients, I've found that there is uncertainty, even shame in the things that one doesn't know, but we have to give ourselves permission to ask questions. After all, it's *your* body." Ask to fully understand the benefits, risks, trade-offs, and alternatives of any major healthcare decision your doctor is advocating. I've learned that one of the key questions to ask in these discussions is: "What would you do if you were in my shoes?" It sounds simple, but it can be both informative and empowering. For understanding lab results, have them explain not just the red flags but also where there may be opportunity for improvement.

4. **Educate yourself from reputable sources.** The goal is to empower yourself to make informed decisions about your own health and the health of your family members. The key to knowing if your source is reputable is to stick to websites of respected and trusted institutions such as Mayo Clinic, the Cleveland Clinic, Johns Hopkins Medicine, the American College of Obstetricians and Gynecologists, and medlineplus .gov (a website produced by the National Institutes of Health). If you look to other sources, such as social media, health-related websites, or newspapers, be sure they link to any studies they discuss. That also applies if you're relying on Google or ChatGPT. As we all know, not everything online is true.

5. **Put your money where your health is.** Health is wealth, and illness is expensive. If you can afford it, pay for the diagnostics to personalize your healthcare needs, the preventive care, the complementary care (acupuncture, chiropractic, massage, or

other modalities that help you feel your best), and the personal trainer who will keep you accountable. Dr. Pham put it succinctly: "If you have disposable income and aren't spending it on your health, then what do you have that money for?"

6. **Stay current on your appointments, shots, screenings, and evaluations.** Yes, it's a lot. And yes, you need to do all the key ones. Refer to the box "Your Healthcare To-Do List" to help you keep track of them all.

Your Healthcare To-Do List

The list below may seem like a lot, but it's about creating a holistic health baseline and, as we live longer, tracking any changes together with your various healthcare professionals. It's also about having the right data to take action before any health problems grow larger. One caveat: Reviewing and interpreting diagnostic results can be daunting and even alarming. Be sure to get your doctor's interpretation of the results. And remember that knowledge really is power. Having the right diagnostic information can help you understand yourself from the inside out and act as an early warning signal of any potential health challenges. Then you have the insights to take action and improve your situation.

Ideally, all this information should be stored in one place for you and all your healthcare providers to access. While this is still somewhat in the future—as different healthcare systems use different electronic healthcare record platforms—we are moving in this direction. In the meantime, ask every provider you see to share lab results and visit notes with your primary care physician.

- Annual physical with primary care physician.
- Annual appointment with a gynecologist (although sometimes your primary care physician can perform your annual pelvic exam—ask to see if you can perhaps consolidate these two appointments).

- Annual in-person skin check with a dermatologist to screen for skin cancer.
- Two dental cleanings per year.
- Biannual mammogram for women fifty and over (this is the current recommendation from the United States Preventive Services Task Force; depending on your family history, risk factors, and breast tissue, you and your doctor may decide to do them more frequently)—whether and how often to get one before you turn fifty is a decision to be made in conversation with your doctor.
- Pap smear and/or a test for the human papilloma virus (HPV, the virus responsible for cervical cancer) at least every three years for women up to age sixty-five, and beyond if you feel it's needed, like I do.
- Annual colon cancer screening for women forty-five and older, whether with a colonoscopy (which requires general anesthesia and a pre-test protocol, which is the worst part) or a Cologuard test (which is best for average-risk individuals and only requires a stool sample); I've done both and they're not fun, but they're important.
- Annual appointment with an ophthalmologist to monitor eye health.
- Baseline bone density evaluation (DEXA scan) at age sixty-five, or at age fifty if you have a higher risk of fracture, although since many women experience a significant decrease in bone density around the age of menopause (more on this in Chapter 8), ask to have it earlier if you want to be proactive. After your first scan, you and your doctor can determine how often to have them going forward—I've done this every so often because I take Synthroid, a prescription medication that treats an underactive thyroid, which can make your bones softer and more vulnerable (and which is also why I am a bit of a fitness fanatic).
- Annual fitness evaluation, performed either by a doctor or by a fitness professional, to assess your cardiovascular capability, muscle and bone strength, gait, and other measures of physical health—you may have to request this from your doctor, who will either perform it or refer you to the right professional.

While the list of our health concerns is long and can grow longer with each passing year, I want to shine a light on just a few health issues that most of us think about, worry about, and may not know how to best navigate as we live longer. We'll take a deep dive into both hormone health and brain health in later chapters, so let's start here by zooming in on the number-one killer of women: heart disease.

HEART HEALTH FOR LIFE

While breast cancer deservedly gets a lot of attention as being a huge health risk for women, heart disease is far and away the number-one killer of women. Sadly, one in three women will die of heart disease, and it often goes undiagnosed.

Cardiologist Dr. Suzanne Steinbaum, whom you first met in Chapter 3, told my writing partner, Kate, that when she was training as a physician twenty years ago, she was in the emergency room and had an aha moment that sealed her future. She recalled:

> A woman was wheeled in, she was about fifty-three years old. She had nausea, vomiting. She was clearly uncomfortable lying on the stretcher. And she was put in the corner with the diagnosis of gastroenteritis or inflammation of the stomach. She proceeded to have a heart attack in the emergency room, under the care of the doctors. I thought to myself, "Women are dying of heart disease. Is everyone seeing what I'm seeing?" And the answer was no, because twenty years ago there was no such thing as women and heart disease. We just didn't know. The research was not done on women.

Oddly, women's and men's heart disease present differently. Dr. Felice Gersh, a board-certified internist and OB/GYN and medical director of the Integrative Medical Group of Irvine, in California, explained the science:

After we go into menopause, our heart mitochondria—the factories of the cell that convert nutrients into energy used throughout the body—stop working properly. Why? Because without enough estradiol [a form of estrogen], mitochondria cannot work properly, and they cannot get rid of the toxic metabolic waste products that they generate during the energy production process. In addition, as we age, the heart loses mitochondria altogether, and the mitochondria that remain don't function well. Simply put: our hearts can run out of gas. You can actually see on an echocardiogram that there's an energy deficiency in a woman's heart. We call that mild diastolic dysfunction—which is something most cardiologists ignore and dismiss with "We see it all the time."

This is a big problem, because, as Gersh said, "When women go into heart failure, it's usually from having mild diastolic dysfunction. Their heart goes into failure because of low energy." Doesn't that feel so apt—that women's hearts work so hard that they can simply run out of energy?

Dr. Steinbaum told me, "In my world there are so many women who've had heart issues that should have been diagnosed and prevented, but they weren't getting regular checkups with their primary care physician." That's one reason it's so important to be consistent with your annual visits to your primary care doctor and keep up with healthy eating, exercise, and sleep—while leaning into your purpose. Remember, every aspect of your ageless aging recipe influences the other.

Blood tests for cholesterol and even C-reactive protein (a marker of inflammation) are standard operating procedure and ordered routinely at an annual visit with your doctor; they are covered by health insurance, including Medicare. Your blood pressure is taken as well. If your annual visit reveals a vulnerability, don't feel defeated. Instead, do something about it. Your doctor should be able to counsel you on lifestyle and pharmaceutical approaches to lower your blood pressure and improve your heart health.

PELVIC HEALTH: A GROWING CONCERN
FOR WOMEN FIFTY AND OVER

The public conversation on pelvic health and incontinence finally seems to be gaining traction, which is a good thing. For years it was considered embarrassing and almost taboo to talk about these things; now there are commercials where women are wearing absorbent underwear and talking openly about wetting their pants. As women live longer, changes in pelvic and urinary health become more common and worrisome. There is an increased risk of weakening in the pelvic floor muscles due to the natural aging process, which can cause urinary and/or fecal incontinence or even pelvic organ prolapse.

Nearly half of women fifty and over say they have urinary leaks ranging from a minor nuisance to a major issue, according to a national poll conducted by the University of Michigan of more than a thousand women between the ages of fifty and eighty. Yet two-thirds of these women hadn't talked to a doctor about it. "Urinary incontinence is a common condition and is usually treatable. It's not an inevitable part of aging and shouldn't be overlooked," said Dr. Carolyn Swenson, a urogynecologist at Michigan Medicine who helped develop and analyze the poll.[2]

It's not just urine that is leaking out of our bodies—the prevalence of pelvic organ prolapse (POP), in which organs such as the uterus or rectum can start pressing into or even peeking out of the vagina, rises significantly as we age. It is expected that 46 percent of American women will experience symptomatic POP—some five million women.[3] We need to open up the conversation to normalize these issues. We all should get regular pelvic exams and any suspicious symptoms should be discussed with a physician.

The good news is that there is a range of successful treatment options for incontinence and prolapse, with new innovations coming down the pike continuously. These include physical therapy (such as Kegel exercises), retraining the bladder, injections of Botox to relax pelvic and/or bladder muscles, sacral nerve stimulation to tone your pelvic floor, urethral bulking agents (injected at the intersection of the bladder and urethra to reduce urine leakage with exercise), and surgical options.

MINIMIZING CHRONIC PAIN

Today, 1.5 billion people worldwide suffer from chronic pain, and 70 percent of those sufferers are women.[4] There isn't a lot of research into the gender differences in the experience of pain, but one seminal study found that women tend to experience pain both more intensely and more frequently than men.[5]

There are many potential ways to alleviate physical pain that can be just as effective as pharmaceuticals while avoiding the host of potential side effects, from constipation to addiction, that come with many prescription pain medications:

- **An anti-inflammatory diet as well as exercise** can ease or eliminate inflammation and its resulting pain.
- **Cryotherapy**, a form of extreme cold treatment, can include things as simple as applying ice packs on a localized portion of the body. Whole-body cryotherapy involves exposing the body to vapors that reach ultra-low temperatures ranging from −150 to −200°F. This temporarily reduces nerve activity and alleviates joint pain and muscle soreness. Basketball stars LeBron James and Steph Curry swear by it. Cryotherapy is popping up in medical spas, high-end fitness clubs, and even longevity clinics all over the country.
- **The Wim Hof Method** is controversial but a social media favorite. It involves breathwork and extreme cold exposure in ice baths combined with mental focus to supercharge the body, gain mastery over your physical and mental states, increase immunity, and decrease the experience of pain. It can be done from the comfort of one's own home by taking ice-cold baths or showers, which sounds terrible to me, but people rave about the results.

- **Infrared saunas,** which are not the same as traditional saunas. They use red and blue light to directly warm the body, whereas a traditional sauna warms the air. A 2022 review of forty-two studies found that infrared therapy is effective in reducing pain levels due to osteoarthritis, fibromyalgia, myofascial pain syndrome, and musculoskeletal injuries.[6] There are countless clinical studies that demonstrate that infrared saunas help combat inflammation, raise immunity, relieve muscle tension, detoxify, and improve quality of sleep. They also have the added benefit of revving up your metabolism, making it easier to lose weight. In total transparency, I am a big fan. Like cryotherapy, this therapy is becoming more available in spas, clinics, and fitness clubs.

- **CBD,** or cannabidiol, is a compound found in cannabis plants. Research has suggested that it interacts with the body's endo-cannabinoid system and may be effective in the management of chronic pain.[7] While CBD has not yet been approved by the FDA for use in treating pain, anecdotal evidence and research support its potential use for this purpose. Kate experiences periodic back pain that tends to flare during stressful periods, and CBD is her go-to form of pain relief—along with a heat pack to the area and craniosacral therapy (a gentle hands-on treatment that aims to restore balance to the flow of cerebral spinal fluid, which lubricates the spine and cranium).

WHEN SHIT HAPPENS...
PRECOVERY TO BOOST HEALING

No matter how many good choices you make and how well you take care of your health, shit happens, especially as we live longer. In fact, aging can sometimes feel like a game of dodgeball, where you find yourself ducking and dodging to avoid catastrophe and stay in the game. In the course of a long life, you are going to get hit with at least a couple of balls that impact your physical health, whether it's a cancer scare, an autoimmune disease, a heart attack, or a joint replacement.

One of the best ways I've found to deal with these curveballs—an approach too few doctors and experts are talking about—is *precovery,* or proactively preparing for the stress of surgery or cancer treatment so you can heal faster, raise your level of immunity and resilience, and even improve your recovery results with the choices you make *before* an event like surgery.

Precovery is a relatively new concept I'd not heard much about until I had to deal with my own unrelenting chronic hip pain and subsequent surgery back in 2019, as I described in the introduction to this book. My surgeon was excellent at surgery but wasn't really familiar with precovery. That put me in the driver's seat. So I did some research and learned that a successful precovery plan works in tandem with your doctor or healthcare provider to go above and beyond traditional protocols to help your body be ready to bounce back better and faster. It's a tool to help you regain some control over your own destiny, which held a lot of appeal to me.

Through my network at Age Wave, I was lucky enough to have access to several top experts who helped me create my own precovery plan. As I shared in the introduction, I cut out foods such as sugar, gluten, and dairy, which can often create an inflammatory response, and I kept exercising, albeit mindfully.

What I didn't share in the introduction is that I was seriously frightened about the surgery, so I also used meditation and affirmations, and I called on my network of friends and family to send positive thoughts my way to optimize my emotional resilience.

In addition, I realized I needed a health advocate in case anything went sideways. I'm not talking about the professional kind, although they certainly can be helpful in a health crisis. I mean a partner, family member, or friend who can advocate for you if and when you are dealing directly with a health issue of any kind and need a person you can rely on to help make smart decisions on your behalf that can impact your future dramatically. I chose my husband, Ken, who is smart and savvy and who loves me. Plus he knows how to navigate the healthcare system. An advocate needs to understand your wants and needs as well as your priorities, so they can make decisions on your behalf if needed. They may also be a helpful sounding board when you're working through your own complex healthcare decisions.

When I finally had the double hip surgery, my surgeon, my anesthesiologist, and the attending nurses all agreed to read the affirmations I provided them with. This was a little corny, I know, but they were happy to do anything that might help. They also told me that other patients were increasingly asking them to do this kind of thing.

I was out of the hospital in one day and up and walking without any assistance, albeit like a duck, two days after surgery with little to no pain.

Precovery also nudged me to create a comprehensive recovery plan so that it was ready to go as soon as I was. I arranged physical therapy well in advance, since the good physical therapy clinics had waiting lists. I also included acupuncture and cryotherapy.

THE FUTURE OF HEALTHCARE: PRECISION MEDICINE

Now that you have some suggestions on how to take more control of your own health through healthcare, let's go a little deeper into personalized, precision medicine, because in terms of medicine and healthcare, one size definitely doesn't fit all. Dr. Pinchas "Hassy" Cohen, professor of gerontology and dean of the USC Leonard David School of Gerontology, explained it to me this way:

> We have to start developing precision approaches that get tailored to each person based on their sex, age, DNA, lifestyle, and various other biomarkers. Chief among these differentiators is sex, as there are plenty of situations where different sexes respond differently to interventions, and honestly, we are just at the beginning of the era where we are exploring these differences in research and practice.

The future of medicine has already begun to appear, allowing healthcare providers to tailor care plans to each individual's genetics and risk factors in what's known as personalized or precision medicine. Dr. Cohen confirmed that precision medicine has already become a staple of oncology. "You don't get diagnosed with cancer today without having a lot of DNA sequencing and molecular analysis to subcategorize your cancer, allowing your physicians to select very precise interventions that fit your particular kind of tumor."

Now the big challenge for the entire field of medicine is to apply that approach to the chronic diseases of aging, including Alzheimer's disease, diabetes, heart disease, Parkinson's, obesity, and frailty. "Currently, we still think of those diseases as a one-size-fits-all situation, and drug companies are searching for a blockbuster drug that will make billions of dollars and everybody will use, but that's so twentieth-century," Cohen said.

Dr. Daniel Kraft, a Stanford- and Harvard-trained physician, scientist, inventor, entrepreneur, innovator, and founder of NextMed Health, which explores convergent, rapidly developing technologies and their potential in biomedicine and healthcare, explained to me how technology is going to play a huge role in the practice of precision medicine: "Part of our future is using AI, big data, and genomics to help pick the right doses of medicines if you need them, or the right screening or other interventions that are going to help you live a longer, healthier life." As an example, let's say you have the BRCA1 or BRCA2 gene, which carries a higher risk of developing breast cancer. You need a different mammogram schedule than someone with no known risk factors. Dr. Kraft continued, "Rather than having the same recommendations that apply to everyone, in the future you and your physician or your healthcare team will have a picture of your genomics and your digital data, possibly collected by wearables or even invisibles, and use that in a much more highly attuned, blended fashion to create a custom healthcare plan for you."

DIAGNOSTIC TESTS: A WINDOW INTO
YOUR HEALTH AND LONGEVITY

The ever-evolving field of diagnostic testing is already beginning to turbocharge precision medicine. I've compiled a menu of advanced diagnostic tests that go beyond the standard blood tests and biometric assessments (such as blood pressure, heart rate, blood/oxygen levels, and weight) that routinely get done at your annual physical. While those standard tests are important, they only begin to scratch the surface when it comes to understanding how your body is functioning and what is needed to prevent or treat disease and help you age more agelessly.

You may have to advocate for many of these tests. Since they are new, many conventional doctors don't include them in their standard workup. You can even order them yourself through Quest Diagnostics, LabCorp, InsideTracker, or other diagnostic providers. Of course, once you get the results, you need an expert to interpret them and help you determine the right actions to take.

Be proactive and discuss these tests with your doctor. Do your research and explain why you want to take them. Know that some of these tests may not be covered by insurance and may be costly. If your doctor doesn't know what to do with the results, find an integrative or functional medicine doctor you trust, either online with telemedicine or near you, to help you understand the results and create a personalized plan based on those results. Telemedicine has empowered us all to find top experts, even if they're many miles away, and they're often covered by insurance, or at least able to be paid for with tax-advantaged funds from a Flexible Spending Account (FSA) or Health Spending Account (HSA). And if you need to pay for these providers out of pocket because they're not covered by your insurance, remember Dr. Christina Pham's question—if you have the money but aren't spending it on your health, what is that money for?

Blood tests
Most of these tests need to be ordered and interpreted by your doctor and can also be reimbursed by Medicare and other insurance. Some you can order yourself.

- **Thyroid testing** to measure thyroid hormones in your blood. The thyroid gland is a master regulator of metabolism and can have far-reaching effects if it is running either too high or too low.
- **Hormone and hormone metabolite panel** to measure your reproductive, stress, and metabolic hormone levels. We'll dive deeper into this in Chapter 8.
- **Heavy metal tests** use either blood or urine to screen for toxic metals such as mercury, lead, and arsenic.
- **Vitamin, mineral, and antioxidant testing** to determine which nutrients you may be deficient in to help guide your eating choices and potential need for supplementation (such as the Genova NutrEval and SpectraCell Laboratories Micronutrient Test Panel). I was experiencing some tingling in my ankle at night, looked up the potential causes, and saw that one of the less scary causes was a B vitamin deficiency. So I had my B vitamin levels and D vitamin levels tested through my doctor, which was covered by insurance. I found that I was, in fact, very low in B vitamins. My doctor recommended I get a B vitamin shot or infusion, which I did, and it corrected the problem quite quickly.
- **Early cancer detection blood tests** screen for up to fifty different kinds of cancers so you can catch them early (especially helpful for cancers that are typically not detected until treatment options are limited, such as ovarian cancer). Companies that offer this include Galleri and OneTest.

Saliva or cheek swab tests

- **Genetic testing** to determine if you have genes or genetic variants that are associated with certain diseases, such as cancer or Alzheimer's.
- **Oral microbiome testing.** Just as your gut is host to trillions of bacteria and fungi, so is your mouth—and this oral ecosystem has a major influence on many other aspects of your health, including dental health, oral health, and even brain health. Available from companies such as Viome and Bristle.

Other tests

- **Biological age testing.** This can be done through blood, urine, or saliva and measures your biological age (in contrast to your chronological age) at a cellular level. Available from Tally Health, Ageless Rx, TruDiagnostic, Elysium Health, myDNAge, and Thorne.

- **Coronary computed tomography angiography (CCTA).** This test uses X-rays to create detailed three-dimensional images of the heart and surrounding structures to assess the risk of coronary artery heart disease, including to detect any narrowing of the artery, as well as any blockages or calcification of the coronary artery walls. It can also be used to assess the condition of the heart muscle and valves, as well as the extent of any damage caused by a heart attack. It provides a baseline for your heart and artery health.

- **Personalized nutrition and lifestyle testing.** These analyze data from DNA tests, blood samples, and an assessment of your lifestyle and nutrition habits to determine your vulnerabilities and develop a plan to optimize your health. Available from InsideTracker.

- **Smartphone app-based tests.** Apps designed to assess symptoms and analyze images make your smartphone able to help you screen for or care for conditions such as cancer (Cancer.Net Mobile), skin diseases (DermAssist), and Alzheimer's disease (MindMate).

- **Wearable activity and sleep trackers.** FitBit started the craze of tracking your activity by wearing a device on your wrist that syncs to your phone, and while they're still at it, they're no longer the only option. The Oura ring (a simple band with multiple sensors that you wear on your finger) and the WHOOP bracelet (which looks like an Apple Watch) track your sleep (how much you got, as well as how much of each type of sleep you got), your heart rate and heart rate variability (a measure of how relaxed and resilient you are), and your overall energy levels—all information that helps you make informed decisions about when to go bed, how much to prioritize stress relief and recovery, and how much activity you need.

- **Full-body MRIs.** These are typically expensive and not covered by insurance, but you can use them to scan for possible early tumors or other structural issues.

CUTTING-EDGE HEALTHCARE DEVELOPMENTS

- **Healthy longevity clinics and medical practices** used to be known as anti-aging medicine, but healthy longevity medicine has come a long way, including a rebranding to *healthy longevity* instead of *anti-aging*. One of the perks of the work I do is that several years ago, my husband, Ken, and I were invited to spend a week at SHA Wellness in Alicante, Spain—a futuristic longevity clinic that combines cutting-edge medical innovations with natural therapies, with a huge emphasis on nutrition. Simply put, the focus there is on helping you live longer, better. The first day there, we were put through a battery of diagnostics. Of course, they found things that needed tweaking. They zeroed in on everything— lifestyle changes, nutrition, supplements and infusions (which most traditional doctors don't recommend), and other therapies and procedures that may help improve health, reduce the risk of age-related diseases, and fine-tune your mental health, cognitive well-being, and physical appearance. Although it was a little overwhelming, I've noticed a growing trend in medical practices and clinics that either specialize in or include a wide range of healthy longevity medicine as part of their offerings.

- **Senolytics** are a broad group of substances that eliminate what's known as senescent cells—cells that no longer function but that don't fully die and get recycled. Senescent cells, which are one of the hallmarks of aging we covered in Chapter 1, can emit inflammatory molecules if they're not removed. The potential good news here is that by removing senescent cells, we could also be removing one of the driving factors of aging. Dr. Cohen told me, "In animal models it appears that that act of eliminating senescent cells results in extension of lifespan as well as the prevention of certain diseases of aging." Dr. James Kirkland, the Noaber Foundation Professor of Aging Research at Mayo Clinic and president of the American Federation for Aging Research, added: "Clinical trials of senolytics are now underway in humans, targeting osteoarthritis, Alzheimer's, and frailty in cancer and bone marrow transplant survivors. It is imperative that we move quickly . . . but cautiously."

Senolytics are probably the most clinically advanced potential interventions for ageless aging because several of them are drugs that are already approved for other things, such as dasatinib, which has been used since the early 2000s to treat some forms of leukemia and lymphoma. Other senolytic compounds are antioxidant nutrients, such as quercetin (found in apples, citrus fruits, and onions) and fisetin (found in strawberries and cucumbers). In the near future, we may be able to take a targeted cocktail of senolytics to remove a certain kind of senescent cell that is contributing to a particular disease (such as macular degeneration or Alzheimer's disease); we may also find a blend that is generally anti-aging. These will have to go through the FDA approval process, so it may take a while.

Metformin is a senolytic drug that inhibits release of harmful products by senescent cells, among other actions. Many longevity hackers are now using it to extend healthy lifespan. It's been used for sixty years to reduce high glucose levels and increase insulin sensitivity in people with diabetes and prediabetes. In those six decades of use, research has observed that diabetics who take metformin enjoy reduced mortality from cardiovascular disease, as well as a lower rate of dementia and stroke. It also seems to help people lose a little weight and help those who are prediabetic avoid or delay developing full diabetes. Animal studies have shown that it extends health in long life.

Since metformin is a widely available drug that helps with so many things that accompany age—and holds the promise of increasing healthy lifespan, although this has not been adequately tested in humans—many healthy people have started to take it off-label solely in the hope of extending their healthy longevity. However, Dr. Pham warned me that it has not been widely tested on women. I tried taking it and had a bad gastrointestinal reaction, so I immediately stopped.

Another potential longevity-enhancing drug that has been adopted by many biohackers is rapamycin, an immunosuppressive drug that has had FDA approval to be used with organ transplant patients since 1999. Rather than acting as a senolytic, which kills senescent cells, rapamycin appears to prevent senescent cells from developing or reduce senescent cells' production of harmful substances. Researchers have discovered that rapamycin extends life expectancy in yeast, worms, and mice. Rapamycin appears to have a similar effect to caloric restriction—it slows down growth, which in turn may slow down aging. But remember, it's immunosuppressive, meaning it can make you more vulnerable to infection. It also happens to cause hyperglycemia (high blood sugar), which over the long term is an invitation to chronic disease. Personally, I'm sitting this one out—although I'm hopeful that we may yet uncover a safe way to harness its life-extending possibilities in a way that also increases healthspan.

- **Focused ultrasound technology.** This could change medical intervention as we know it. It is a noninvasive treatment that uses sound waves to treat targeted areas in the body with no needles, cutting, radiation, or anesthesia required. That means no hospital stays, no bleeding, and no risk of infection. Focused ultrasound has had FDA approval as a treatment for uterine fibroids since 2003, and since then has earned it for seven more uses, including bone cancer treatment and Parkinson's-related tremors and other movement—and its use in breast cancer treatment is nearing FDA approval at this writing.

  Dr. Suzanne LeBlang explained focused ultrasound as multiple sound waves sent into the body that converge at a specific target, "like shining a group of flashlights inside the body and then, at the point where all the beams converge, you can make a lot of things happen." When used on tumors or fibroids, focused ultrasound heats the targeted tissue and kills the cells, so the tumor or fibroid is destroyed. It's also used to deliver medicine directly to the tissue that needs it—such as directing a chemotherapy agent directly to the site of a tumor, or even penetrating the blood-brain barrier to get medicine into a precise location in the brain, which has multiple possibilities for treating brain tumors as well as neurodegenerative diseases such as Alzheimer's disease and other dementias as well as Parkinson's.

Some medical centers, such as Stanford, Brigham and Women's Hospital in Boston, and Mayo Clinic, are already using focused ultrasound. You can also visit the Focused Ultrasound Foundation website (www.fusfoundation.org/) to find a treatment center. This website will also tell you which clinical trials you may be eligible for. What's exciting to me about focused ultrasound is not only that it improves treatment outcomes, but also that it is less invasive, less painful, and less likely to create a cascade of unpleasant side effects. LeBlang agrees it holds great promise: "I think focused ultrasound gives us all tremendous hope that we are going to live longer, and we're going to live better."

- **Virtual medicine.** Telemedicine has been around for a while and was boosted by the pandemic, when we were all forced to stay home. This trend will only grow stronger, and many appointments will be able to be conducted via video technology. It also potentially gives you access to specialists who are on the other side of the country or the other side of the globe. As I write this, Samsung has just released TVs with a built-in telemedicine app that claims to connect you with a doctor within sixty seconds; in addition to conducting a remote exam, these doctors can call in prescriptions for you. Samsung has also debuted a Health Monitor app included on their newest TVs that uses a camera (that's not built into the TV, yet—you have to have a compatible one plugged into the set) and technology known as remote photoplethysmography to assess tiny color changes on your face as you breathe to measure vital signs including heart rate, respiration rate, and blood oxygen saturation.

- **Smart toilets.** You can tell a lot about your health from molecules that are present in your urine (such as whether you are in ketosis, whether there is too much sugar in your urine, your hydration level, where you are in your menstrual cycle if you still have one) and your stool (the status of your microbiome, whether you have genetic changes that indicate you're at greater risk of colon cancer, whether you have certain infections). Rather than buying at-home test kits or collecting samples and sending them to a lab, your toilet may soon be able to do an assessment for you. A company called Withings has developed a device called the U-SCAN—a palm-sized disc that sits inside your toilet and analyzes your urine—and I'll bet other companies will soon follow suit.

- **Invisibles.** Currently, we have wearables that monitor our vital signs, but soon you won't even need to wear something on your body, Dr. Daniel Kraft tells me. "The camera on your laptop or smartphone will soon be able to detect your heart rate, blood pressure, oxygen saturation, maybe even heart rate variability. So, while you're on a Zoom call, your vitals could be collected, or the camera could be analyzing your face, your eyes, and your voice, as changes in your voice can indicate signs of early neurologic disorder like Parkinson's disease, or whether you have heart disease, or if that cough is a common cold or the flu or croup or COVID."

HEALTHCARE: WHERE TO BEGIN

**If you do one thing: Ask your doctor to test for heavy metals
when ordering your annual blood test**

You need to confirm whether this is covered by your insurance, but I strongly recommend this screening, especially if you eat a lot of sushi. I had this done through my doctor, found that my heavy metals were too high, and made changes in my diet. I also added cilantro and chlorella to my diet, which are natural chelators, and was able to rid myself of the buildup of toxic metals, which can cause serious health problems including fatigue, memory loss, kidney damage, and a higher risk of cancer.

If you're a total beginner: Find a primary care doctor and a gynecologist you can trust and relate to, and schedule your annual exams

Some primary care physicians do gynecologic exams, which eliminates one doctor visit. Here's another tip: schedule your next appointment before you leave the office, so that you don't have to remember to do it a year later.

If you are already on top of your healthcare and are ready to take it to the next level: Take advantage of at-home diagnostics regularly

In order to be the CEO of your own healthcare, you need to know your own body. There are a handful of biometrics that provide insight into your general state of health. Luckily, you can make at-home testing a regular part of your routine. Recording your results in a notebook will help you objectively assess your trends over time.

- **Weigh yourself regularly.** Yes, I know we hate the scale, but it provides vital information. Long-term changes in weight could be an indicator of a health problem—although it's important to note that your weight naturally fluctuates daily and a difference of a few pounds from morning to night is not something to stress over. This isn't about knowing how skinny or fat you are—it's about monitoring the trend of your weight.
- **Take your blood pressure regularly.** High blood pressure or hypertension is a condition in which the pressure of blood against the artery walls is too high. It's a risk factor for heart disease and stroke. Taking your blood pressure at home with a blood pressure cuff is easy to do and will give you an indication of your heart health. Blood pressure cuffs can be purchased online and

are generally under $100. In general, healthy blood pressure is considered to be 120/80 mmHg or less.

- **Measure your blood oxygen level regularly.** Use a pulse oximeter, an inexpensive device you can find online or at your local drugstore.
- **Test your gut microbiome.** Do this twice annually, with one of the services listed earlier in the chapter. These test results are easy to interpret and include a list of your superfoods, foods to enjoy, and foods to avoid. And, of course, the services all sell supplements based on your test results.
- **Test your biological age.** Do this annually, with one of the services listed earlier in this chapter, so that you can assess how your ageless aging recipe is impacting your rate of aging. At this writing, longevity pioneer Dr. David Sinclair has created Tally Health, which is membership-based; it measures your biological age with an easy mouth swab and then makes recommendations to help you live longer, better.

AGELESS AGING HACKS TO OPTIMIZE YOUR RELATIONSHIP WITH HEALTHCARE

Get to know your community pharmacist

Katy Votava, who has a PhD in health economics and nursing and is president and founder of Goodcare, knows how to navigate the healthcare system and Medicare with finesse. She is a big advocate of having all your prescriptions filled at a community pharmacy (as opposed to a big-box store or through online ordering). "Your community pharmacist is an overlooked healthcare resource," she told me. "When you get all your prescriptions through them, they will automatically check to see how one drug might interact with your other medications. They can also help you work with your insurance provider to get more of your prescriptions covered—or find a generic that has a lower cost." More and more, pharmacies are also doing immunizations and other quick visits that don't cost extra, and that really helps.

Invest in a concierge doctor

Following Dr. Pham's advice to invest in your health and healthcare, you may want to consider finding a concierge doctor. This isn't a new idea, but it's definitely gaining traction as frustrations with the healthcare system build for both patients and doctors. Concierge practices limit the number of patients they take on so their doctors can spend more time with patients and provide more personalized care. The benefits can be enormous: greater access to care (you can often get same-day or next-day appointments—and spend more time with your doctor at every appointment), more in-depth medical consultation, and less stress and frustration with the healthcare system. And they usually have more leverage with specialists they recommend to you, which can also mean quicker appointments with those trusted professionals. Concierge medicine comes with a price tag that varies from region to region, but in most of the country, it can be worth the investment and might even save you money in the long run by emphasizing wellness and preventive care.

Try NAD+ with a "before" and "after" biological age test to check its impact

Nicotinamide adenine dinucleotide, or NAD+, is used by longevity hackers at the cutting edge, like David Sinclair and Dave Asprey. It is an essential enzyme that plays a role in an array of cellular and neuronal functions, as well as inflammation and circadian rhythm—and it decreases with age.[8] This decline is believed to play a role in the development of wrinkles, neurodegenerative diseases, and metabolic disorders. And certain evidence-based longevity hacks—including exercise and caloric restriction—are believed to extend lifespan because they increase NAD+.[9] Most of the studies on increasing NAD+ levels by supplementing with nicotinamide mononucleotide (NMN, a precursor to NAD+) or nicotinamide riboside (NR, another precursor) have been conducted on mice, but those have shown that it prevents or delays the development of age-related disease, extending healthspan, as well as preventing age-related weight gain, improving insulin sensitivity, mitigating age-related changes to gene expression, and improving memory in animal models of Alzheimer's disease.[10] A 2023 randomized controlled trial gave eighty healthy middle-aged adults either a placebo or 300 mg, 600 mg, or 900 mg of NMN for sixty days. All groups who received some level of NMN had increased NAD+ levels, compared to the control group and to themselves at the start of the trial. There were no adverse events or safety issues reported. All groups who received some dosage of NMN achieved significantly higher walking distances during a six-minute walking test (the 600 mg and 900 mg groups had the longest walking distances). I take NMN daily and feel no different than I did before I started taking it. However, I have seen marked improvements in some of my diagnostic tests, including in my glucose levels, so I keep taking it.[11]

Take nitric oxide supplements

While there aren't a lot of hard-and-fast supplement rules except to know that most are not FDA approved, one supplement you might not have heard of but should consider taking is nitric oxide. I learned about it when I attended the 27th Annual A4M (American Academy of Anti-Aging Medicine) World Congress, a premier longevity conference attended by thousands of doctors and health practitioners involved in longevity medicine, functional and integrative medicine, and adjacent fields. There was a lot of buzz about nitric oxide and its benefits as you age.

By the time you hit fifty, your nitric oxide levels can drop by 35 percent compared to those of your twenty-year-old self. Nitric oxide is a vasodilator, which means it relaxes the inner muscles of blood vessels, causing them to widen. As a result, nitric oxide increases blood flow to your extremities and lowers blood pressure—this is why children's hands and feet are always so warm, while older adults' appendages tend to be colder. Nitric oxide also has an effect on inflammation, which generally increases with the years, and on the occurrence of pain, making it a valuable tool in fighting pain, including arthritis pain.

Although exercise can help improve the functioning of the nitric oxide molecule in your body—as can foods rich in nitric oxide like spinach and beets—a nitric oxide supplement has no known negative side effects. You can assess your nitric oxide levels with saliva test strips that you can find online or in many drugstores. Many available supplements come with a test strip so you can measure your levels to establish a baseline and then track your improvements.

If you take a statin drug to lower cholesterol and experience muscle weakness, try CoQ10

I have high cholesterol. Although I haven't eaten meat in forty years, I exercise regularly, and I minimize dairy, sugar, and gluten, I have a genetic predisposition for it. So, my doctor recommended I take a statin to control my cholesterol level. However, I started to experience muscle weakness soon after starting with the statin. I called my doctor to discuss this, and she recommended I take the supplement coenzyme Q10 (CoQ10), which could eliminate this side effect. This is because coenzyme Q10 is used by every cell in the body to produce energy, and statins reduce the mechanism that produces both cholesterol and coenzyme Q10. With less coenzyme Q10 on hand, it's theorized that your muscles can have less access to energy, with weakness and soreness as a result—so theoretically, adding more coenzyme Q10 could remedy this occasional side effect of statins (although no large trials have found that it has more of a beneficial impact than a placebo). I tried the supplement. Guess what? It worked!

8

◆

HORMONES ARE YOUR FRENEMIES

There are two sides to every coin, and women's reproductive hormones are no exception. Many scientists believe that female hormones are, in part, responsible for giving us women our longevity bonus—the fact that we outlive men by an average of six years. Endogenous estrogen (that is, the estrogen our bodies make) in particular appears to have protective properties that may explain why we often get chronic degenerative diseases such as heart disease, high blood pressure, and stroke about ten years later than men.

As our ovaries produce less estrogen, its protective benefits decline—and that's part of the reason women tend to get sicker than men in the second half of life. "The onset of menopause is associated with increasing our risk of cardiovascular disease, osteoporosis, neurodegenerative diseases, and autoimmune disease," said Jennifer Garrison, PhD, assistant professor at the Buck Institute for Research on Aging. In this way, female hormones are like the best friend and protector who disappears just when you need her the most, hence the term "frenemies" in this chapter's title.

On top of that naturally occurring disadvantage, for centuries female hormones have been deemed taboo. In the scientific realm, our hormones have been considered "confounding factors," and thus women have largely not been included in research studies until very recently.

Even the research that has been conducted on postmenopausal women has often suffered from design flaws and been misinterpreted, which has led to millions of women being steered away or outright denied the care they need.

Fortunately, things are changing: "There's a moment happening right now which is a sea change in that we're having a societal dialogue around women's hormones," Garrison told me. "I think it's partly because this generation of women who are coming up against perimenopause and menopause, instead of just quietly accepting the status quo, are saying, 'No thank you. No way. No one ever told me about this.'"

Understanding your hormones, the way they fluctuate in midlife, and what you can do about it is an essential ingredient in ageless aging. Knowledge can be a superpower, and my aim in this chapter is to make you a superhero.

YOUR OVARIES ARE OLDER THAN YOU ARE

Paradoxically, menopause is not really about the decline in reproductive hormones. Yes, that's a huge factor, but hormone levels decline only because the ovaries are aging rapidly—about two and a half times the rate of all other tissues. This ovarian aging is technically called ovarian senescence. "By the time a woman is in her mid-30s, when the rest of her body is functioning at peak performance, her ovaries are already considered geriatric by the medical community," explained Garrison. (If you had children past age thirty-five, as I did, now you know—your pregnancy wasn't considered geriatric because *you* were old, it was because your ovaries were.)

However, there is an upside to ovarian senescence from a research perspective, as Garrison explained. "Ovaries are a gift to the longevity research community, because it gives you a human model for accelerated aging, one that's testable, and one that can be used in clinical trials." Wouldn't it be a mind-bender if women's ovaries, which had caused us to be left out of the research conversation for so long, actually launched women to the forefront of scientific exploration?

Menopause Glossary

BHRT. Bioidentical hormone replacement therapy. The most commonly prescribed bioidentical hormones are estrogen, progesterone, and testosterone. Some bioidentical hormones are approved by the FDA and made by pharmaceutical companies in standardized dosages. Others are made to order by a pharmacy that compounds the hormones in amounts that are specific to each patient, but most physicians will advise against using these except in rare circumstances since FDA-approved treatments are considered safer, with more consistent dosing.

Estrogen. This is an umbrella term describing a family of hormones that your body produces at different times in your life. Estradiol is the form of estrogen manufactured during your reproductive years, estriol is the primary form of estrogen you make when you are pregnant, and estrone is what you make after menopause. Of these, estradiol is the most potent form. Importantly, estrogen plays a role in managing levels of cholesterol, blood sugar, bone mass, muscle mass, and collagen, as well as cardiovascular and brain health. It really is like the most popular girl in class—friends with everyone.

HRT. Hormone replacement therapy; the terms HT and MHT have largely replaced HRT since HT's end goal is not to replace your hormones—it is to treat symptoms of menopause.

HT. Hormone therapy. The term refers to prescribing either estrogen alone, in the form of estradiol or conjugated equine estrogens (CEE, sold under the name Premarin), or in conjunction with progesterone, in the form of the bioidentical progesterone or the synthetic progestin.

Menopause. The point in time when it's been one year since your last period. On average women are between fifty and fifty-two when this happens.

MHT. Menopausal hormonal therapy. This is the same as HT and the terms can be used interchangeably.

Perimenopause. The time when your ovaries start producing less consistent levels of reproductive hormones and your period gets erratic. "It's like your ovaries are on one day and off the next, and these fluctuating levels can trigger a lot of concerning symptoms," explained Dr. Carol Kuhle, director of the Menopause and Women's Sexual Health Clinic at Mayo Clinic. It can last anywhere from a few months to over a decade, but on average, women experience perimenopausal symptoms for three to four years.

Postmenopause. Everything that comes after that one-year anniversary of your last period.

Premenopause. When you are cycling regularly—or at least, regularly for you.

Progesterone. The hormone progesterone, which declines with age, is best known for making sure the uterine lining is ripe for a potential pregnancy and helping an early pregnancy remain viable. But it also works throughout the body in concert with estrogen premenopausally to protect bone health, soothe the nervous system, and protect the brain.[1]

Testosterone. Typically testosterone is thought of as a male hormone, but women make it, too, in their ovaries as well as their adrenal glands. It plays a role in libido, in building and maintaining muscle and bone mass, and in the formation of estrogen. While we don't lose testosterone completely as we transition through menopause (both the ovaries and the adrenals continue to make it), it does continue to decline slowly over time starting in your thirties.

SYMPTOMS OF PERIMENOPAUSE AND MENOPAUSE

While we're waiting for ovaries to lead the way in longevity research, we have some very real—and at times debilitating—symptoms created by their senescence to reckon with. Here are the typical symptoms of peri- and postmenopause broken out by category.

Menstrual

These are typically some of the first perimenopausal symptoms to show up.

- Skipped periods (although pregnancy is still possible)
- Shorter cycles
- Spotting
- More intense bleeding

Vasomotor

"Vasomotor" means anything that causes the contraction or dilation of blood vessels; in menopause, vasomotor symptoms are hot flashes and night sweats. While the term refers to the cardiovascular system, the effects of vasomotor-related symptoms extend to the brain. "Vasomotor symptoms are more than just a bad feeling—some studies have looked at MRIs of the brain in women who have untreated vasomotor symptoms and found changes in the brain," Dr. Kuhle told me.

- Palpitations
- Hot flashes
- Chills
- Night sweats, which can impact your sleep and negatively affect your cognitive function

Brain and mood

Perimenopause is a true mind-body issue—it can impact cognition, memory, and mood, in such a way that you may not even feel like yourself. "I think every woman in her forties or fifties who has been happily married and now finds herself contemplating divorce should consult with a menopause-savvy physician about whether hormonal fluctuations could be playing a role, because there's such intense change that happens for women that goes unchecked as a potential medical issue," said Dr. Krista Ramonas, a physician board-certified in longevity medicine and CEO of The Lab by Custom Med in San Francisco.

- Brain fog
- Memory problems
- Irritability
- Stress and anxiety
- Feeling down

Sleep

Part of the sleep difficulties that are common in menopause are tied to vasomotor symptoms—it's hard to sleep when you're overheated. But part of the difficulties are due to the fact that peri- and postmenopausal women are more prone to chronic activation of the sympathetic nervous system, which rules the fight-or-flight response. That makes it harder to relax enough to sleep deeply.

- Difficulty falling asleep
- Middle-of-the-night awakenings

Structural

Joints and bones have receptors for estrogen. In joints, estrogen has an anti-inflammatory effect, so when it declines, joints can get swollen, stiff, and sore. In bones, estrogen acts as a regulator of the rate of bone turnover; without it, bones can lose density and strength.

- Joint pain
- Thinning bones
- Thinning hair
- Dry skin
- Change in breast shape and fullness

Sexual health

Menopause has a big impact on sexual health—one we need to talk about openly. Because estrogen protects vaginal tissue, you can experience physical changes that make sex feel less good (and can contribute to urinary incontinence as well as urinary tract and bladder infections). Sex can be a major way we feel that all-important connection to another human, so if you are having sexual concerns, talking with your clinician is a good idea. It's also a great stress reliever and, honestly, who couldn't use more pleasure and playfulness in their lives?

- Drop in libido and sexual satisfaction
- Vaginal dryness
- Painful intercourse
- Urinary incontinence
- Bladder infections

ASSESSING YOUR SYMPTOMS:
THE MENOPAUSE RATING SCALE

The Menopause Rating Scale was designed in the 1990s as a way for women to objectively assess the severity of their perimenopause and menopausal symptoms. When used as an assessment before and after an intervention, it can serve as a way to gauge the effectiveness of any treatments. To use it, check a box next to each common symptom; if you don't experience that symptom, check None. At the end, add up your scores. A score of 0–4 is minimal, 5–8 is mild, 9–15 is moderate, and anything over 16 is severe. For an online version, visit www .menopause-rating-scale.info.

Symptom	None 0	Mild 1	Moderate 2	Severe 3	Extreme 4
Hot flashes, sweating					
Heart palpitations, racing or skipping a heartbeat					

Symptom	None 0	Mild 1	Moderate 2	Severe 3	Extreme 4
Sleep problems (difficulty falling asleep, middle of the night wakefulness, waking up early)					
Blue mood (feeling down, sad, on the verge of tears, lack of drive, mood swings)					
Irritability (feeling nervous, stressed, aggressive, short-tempered)					
Anxiety (feeling panicky, worried, restless)					
Physical and mental exhaustion (memory problems, difficulty concentrating, forgetfulness, fatigue)					
Sexual problems (lack of desire, painful or uncomfortable intercourse, decrease in satisfaction)					
Bladder problems (incontinence, increased urge to urinate, difficulty urinating, bladder infections)					

Symptom	None 0	Mild 1	Moderate 2	Severe 3	Extreme 4
Vaginal changes (dryness, burning, discomfort, or pain during sex)					
Joint and muscular discomfort (joint pain, aches, rheumatoid complaints)					

UNPACKING MHT: THE GOOD, THE BAD, AND THE MISGUIDED

There's good news and bad news when it comes to alleviating the symptoms of menopause. The good news is that the gold standard for treatment of menopausal symptoms has been in use, with FDA approval, for decades. It's menopausal hormone therapy, or HT, and it consists of prescribing estrogen, progesterone, and sometimes even testosterone to treat symptoms of menopause.

The bad news is that, thanks largely to the misinterpretation of results of one poorly designed study that got a lot of attention in 2002, HT is misunderstood and miscommunicated by many doctors—even gynecologists—to their patients. As a result, it unfortunately is no longer the go-to standard of care. A 2021 survey by the company Bonafide found that 73 percent of postmenopausal women were experiencing menopausal symptoms but not treating them, and 65 percent said they would not consider using HT. That's how pervasive the fear of HT has become.[2] Looking at how we got here is an eye-opener.

HT was a standard of care for decades, ever since the FDA approved conjugated equine estrogens—that's an estrogen derived from horse urine, which is still in use and sold under the brand name Premarin (which is short for "pregnant mares urine")—in 1942. Our understanding of HT wasn't without its hiccups. For example, in 1975, the medical establishment realized that prescribing estrogen alone increased the risk of endometrial cancer, but quickly corrected course and began prescribing a progestogen along with estrogen to alleviate that risk. (In a premenopausal woman, progestogens prevent the lining of the uterus from ripening, so when taken after menopause, they protect the uterine lining from experiencing growth that can lead to cancer.)

HT was working to do more than merely alleviate hot flashes and other symptoms: a 1991 observational study on nearly fifty thousand nurses found that postmenopausal women on HT had a 50 percent lower risk of coronary heart disease than women who were not taking hormones.[3] However, that same year, the National Institutes of Health started tracking the health outcomes of nearly 160,000 women who were randomized into taking HT or not taking HT. That study, known as the Women's Health Initiative or WHI, was designed to follow the women for as long as fifteen years. But in 2002, the WHI steering committee abruptly called a halt to the study, saying that what they had actually found was an increase in the risk of both heart disease and breast cancer in women who were taking HT. In reality, the risk of developing breast cancer rose just a tiny amount—from 2.33 percent to 2.94 percent. The mainstream media, however, reported this as an increase in risk of 26 percent. While that percentage was accurate, it was 26 percent of a very small number. (To help put these numbers in context, smoking skyrockets the risk of cancer by a whopping 2,600 percent.) The coverage was misinterpreted and, not surprisingly, sowed widespread fear of HT.

Not only were the risks distorted, but the study design had major flaws. Namely, it mostly included women who were already sixty or older, more than ten years from menopause, and taking hormones for the first time. The risk of cancer and heart disease naturally rises with age, muddling the actual benefits of HT itself. It turns out that the age of initiation of HT matters. For women who were fifty to fifty-nine in the WHI, they in fact did not have significantly increased risk of cardiovascular disease, even up until eighteen years post-randomization. So, starting HT early in menopause appears to be safer than later in menopause. In addition, the hormones used in the study were *synthetic* hormones, not bioidentical hormones.

"Bioidentical means the hormone is the same chemical compound that your ovary makes," Dr. Kuhle explained to me, and that is what women should be using. Why? Because if you modify a chemical compound just a tiny bit, it can have a tremendously different effect. For example, water is H_2O. If you add one extra oxygen molecule, it becomes H_2O_2, which is hydrogen peroxide—not something that's going to quench your thirst.

The WHI used conjugated equine estrogens from the urine of pregnant horses, not estradiol, which is the same chemical compound made by the ovaries. As Dr. Gersh explained, "A pregnant horse has very different estrogen than a reproductive age woman."

The form of progestogen that the WHI used was called medroxy-progesterone (known as Provera), technically a member of a family of chemicals called progestins that are able to bind to progesterone receptors. "Progestins are technically an endocrine disruptor for pro-gesterone," Dr. Gersh explained.

One more weakness in the WHI study: they administered estrogen in pill form. "An estrogen pill is metabolized through the liver, which can increase the risk for stroke," Dr. Kuhle explained. With a patch or other non-oral estradiol formulation, the estradiol is absorbed through your skin, bypassing the liver. That's why today it is common—but not necessarily standard—practice to prescribe estradiol (the bioidentical form of estrogen) in a transdermal application, such as a patch or gel.

Once the WHI bomb exploded, as reported by the *New York Times Magazine* in a 2023 cover story, "panic set in; in one year, the number of prescriptions plummeted. Hormone therapy carries risks, to be sure, as do many medications that people take to relieve serious discomfort, but dozens of studies since 2002 have provided reassurance that for healthy women under sixty whose hot flashes are troubling them, the benefits of taking hormones outweigh the risks." (The title of this article summed it up succinctly: "Women Have Been Misled About Menopause.")[4]

The WHI did teach us helpful things. Later analyses of the WHI data found that women who begin HT *after* age sixty have a small increase in heart disease risk, and that risk becomes significant in women who start after seventy.[5] "There's a line in the sand around age sixty," Dr. Kuhle told me. However, *if you are already on HT, as I have been, your risk of heart disease goes up because of age, but is likely not related to HT.* On the positive side, it also showed that women on HT had a significant reduction in the risk of bone fractures and type 2 diabetes (compared to placebo), and that women on estrogen alone had a lower risk of breast cancer or mortality related to breast cancer (compared to placebo).[6]

SEPARATING FACT FROM FICTION

The Women's Health Initiative study did lead to some important takeaways:

- FDA-approved bioidentical hormone therapy has some benefits over synthetic hormones. That means using estradiol and progesterone. Yet some insurance companies, doctors, and pharmacies will try to give you the synthetics, so *you need to ask for bioidenticals.*
- You likely want your estradiol to come in a non-oral formulation such as a patch.
- It's better to start HT early, certainly before age sixty or within ten years of your last menstrual period.

Beyond that, you may also want to consider taking testosterone, particularly if you are struggling with low libido and having difficulty maintaining and building muscle.

Many functional medicine and longevity medicine doctors use a compounding pharmacy to make HT customized to your precise health and genetic profile. Dr. Kuhle said she discourages compounding because it's not regulated, so you don't always know what you're getting, and it can be expensive. It is also not supported by medical evidence. "We avoid compounding, except for testosterone, because there is no FDA-approved bioidentical option currently for women. In that instance [when prescribing testosterone], we'll follow their testosterone levels to make sure they're not getting too much," Dr. Kuhle said.

Timing is also a variable that you can discuss with your doctor, particularly when it comes to progesterone. My doctor had me taking progesterone every day of the month because it helps support better sleep, while some clinicians, including Dr. Gersh, recommend taking it only two weeks out of every month because it more closely mimics your body's premenopausal flow of hormones. "Progesterone is only being released during the second half of the menstrual cycle," Dr. Gersh told me.

Two prominent studies on the effectiveness of HT that have been conducted since the WHI study—the KEEPS study and the ELITE study—tested estradiol and pulsed progesterone (which means participants took progesterone for only two weeks out of the month) and found that women who started the therapy within a few years of menopause experienced a significant reduction in symptoms related to menopause and sexual health, and enjoyed improvement in cardiovascular health with no increased risk of clotting events, such as deep vein thrombosis.[7]

Kate and I both tried taking the higher dose of progesterone in a pulsed approach, but noticed that on the days when we weren't taking it, we didn't sleep as well, and Kate noticed that she got more headaches. We're all very unique individuals, reacting to hormones in different ways, so you may have to experiment to find the right approach for you. (Now we take a smaller dosage every day.)

The final thing to consider is your goals for HT. Most of us are trying to remedy our menopausal symptoms, for which a very low dosage of estrogen is typically prescribed. However, there are those who want to take it further, with the goal of extended longevity. If that's the case, consider what Dr. Gersh told me: "You have to reframe your thinking and aim to restore physiologic amounts of hormones in a physiologic rhythm. That means a higher dose of estrogen than is generally prescribed to manage symptoms of menopause, and a higher dose of progesterone taken for only a portion of the month." While I'm not advocating this, and it's not in line with evidence-based practice or clinical guidelines, this is a path that some are taking.

CONFUSION AND MISINFORMATION
STILL LEAD TO MISGUIDANCE

Unfortunately, many OB/GYNs—the type of doctors most women are talking to about their hormonal health—are still resistant to, or downright dismissive of, prescribing hormone therapy. And much of this resistance is still lingering as a direct result of the Women's Health Initiative study.

While all doctors must practice medicine with a sensitivity to caution, not only because they have people's lives in their hands, but also because they rightly fear getting sued, OB/GYNs are extra-susceptible to liability concerns because they deal with pregnancy and birth. I can't blame them for wanting to be cautious. And if they went to medical school after 2002, when the WHI study came out, they likely learned that the risks outweigh the benefits when it comes to HT. They are simply practicing medicine as they were taught . . . which was based on faulty, outdated information. But there's too much at stake to continue to dismiss HT on a broad scale.

THE SERIOUS HEALTH RISKS OF MENOPAUSE
GO FAR BEYOND QUALITY OF LIFE

Peri- and postmenopausal symptoms can be unpleasant, but that's just the tip of the iceberg. To understand the role of hormones in your ageless aging—and why you might want to ask your doctor about bioidentical HT—consider the widespread effects of what Dr. Gersh describes as "an accumulation of deficiencies initiated by the lack of hormones triggered by the declining function of the ovaries."

Let's take a quick tour through the many systems, organs, and tissues impacted.

- **Brain health and cognitive function.** Declining estrogen is associated with a decrease in memory and cognitive function and an increase in risk of dementia. Thankfully, HT appears to counter these declines—a 2020 review of twenty-one studies concluded that "estrogen replacement therapy significantly decreased the risk of onset and/or development of Alzheimer's Disease."[8]

- **Liver.** The loss of hormonal homeostasis can trigger the liver to make too much cholesterol and triglycerides, and to become insulin resistant.[9] In addition to jeopardizing heart and metabolic health, this can lead the liver to store excess glucose as fat, and one in four people worldwide now has metabolic dysfunction-associated steatotic liver disease (MASLD). The liver is a key support player for the rest of the body. You want it in good shape.

- **Bone density.** "When you start to go through perimenopause, you can have a precipitous loss of bone," Dr. Kuhle said. Bone loss means increased risk of fracture and increased vulnerability to falling, but hormone replacement can help.

- **The microbiome, gut wall integrity, and inflammation.** There is a symbiotic relationship between your microbiome and estrogen— your gut flora produce bioavailable estrogen, and when estrogen is low it can disrupt the balance between good gut bugs and bad. This imbalance can contribute to intestinal permeability, which allows particles from the GI tract to leak into the bloodstream where they can trigger an immune response that may go overboard and cause harm—intestinal permeability has been associated with conditions such as IBS and celiac disease.[10] (Intestinal permeability is sometimes referred to as leaky gut, a condition that, it should be said, tends to be identified as a root cause of autoimmune conditions by health influencers and viewed with skepticism by medically trained doctors. But women are four times more likely to have an autoimmune condition than men—it seems reasonable to hypothesize that estrogen may be playing a role.[11])

- **Metabolic health and belly fat/waist circumference.** Estrogen has a broad impact on metabolism—it helps burn fat, facilitates the formation of insulin, and regulates blood sugar. Researchers have called its various metabolic roles "fairly close to a recipe for preventing the development of metabolic syndrome."[12]

- **Muscle tone.** Declining testosterone levels contribute to reduced muscle mass—a factor in fall risk and frailty as we age and an impediment to both healthspan and lifespan. Yet few doctors are prescribing testosterone replacement for women, in no small part because there is no FDA-approved form of testosterone replacement for women.

- **Mitochondrial function.** Estradiol is essential for mitochondrial function. Mitochondria are the organelles within your cells that are responsible for producing the energy that fuels nearly every bodily process. "Without enough estradiol, mitochondria cannot get rid of the metabolic waste products that they create as a byproduct of manufacturing energy," Dr. Gersh said. These waste products are poison, and over time their buildup will impair the mitochondria's ability to produce energy—not something you want if you're planning to live well for a long time.

- **Circadian clock.** "Many postmenopausal women have dysregulated appetite and circadian rhythms, because estrogen also regulates the master clock in the brain," Dr. Gersh said. "It's almost like they're living jet-lagged lives—they want to stay up, and they want to eat all night long."

HEALTH RISKS THAT MAY
SUGGEST HT IS RIGHT FOR YOU

Here's a simple list of risks to help you assess how likely a candidate you are for HT.

- Early hip fractures in your family.
- Dementia in your family.
- Cardiovascular disease in your family.
- A diagnosis of osteopenia.

- Vasomotor symptoms.
- Decreasing metabolic health (increase in blood sugar and waist circumference).
- A high score on your Menopause Rating Scale.

As you can see from this list, family history is important. If you have a parent or grandparent who suffered from dementia and/or osteoporosis, and you are experiencing menopausal symptoms, the benefits of HT may likely outweigh any risks.

This is the case for Kate, who initially talked to her OB/GYN about HT to treat her night sweats (which were interrupting her sleep) and painful intercourse when she was fifty and had just passed the one-year anniversary of her last period. But her doctor, who attended medical school after the WHI study came out, waved her off because, she said, the risks of heart disease and breast cancer were too high. But no one in Kate's family has ever had breast cancer or heart disease—and both her grandmothers had dementia. In addition, Kate was diagnosed with osteopenia. So she visited the Menopause Society website (www.menopause.org) to find a menopause-certified doctor, who put her on an estradiol patch with oral progesterone. (Because there are so few menopause-certified doctors out there, Kate spent several weeks on a waiting list for an appointment—she called the office every other week and finally managed to get in when someone else canceled their appointment at the last minute.)

In general, it's better to start HT before you are sixty; how long you stay on it after that is a discussion for you and your (hopefully menopause-certified) doctor. According to the experts I spoke to, the earlier you start talking to your doctor about your symptoms and potential treatments for them, the better. (And if your doctor dismisses you, start your search for a menopause- and HT-savvy physician now.)

The bottom line on HT is that there is no one-size-fits-all approach. Every clinician I spoke with told me that they need to customize hormone therapy based on individual symptoms and health risks.

HEALTH RISKS THAT SUGGEST
THAT HT MAY BE TOO RISKY

All this being said, HT is not appropriate for everyone. The following considerations need to be taken into account.

- Premenopausal breast or other hormone-related cancer in you or your family. If you or your mother, sister, or aunt has or has had a hormone-related cancer, such as breast, uterine, ovarian, or endometrial, taking estradiol may increase your risk of developing cancer. For this reason, you need to have a candid discussion with your doctor about your cancer risk and follow their orders.
- More than ten years since menopause without having used HT. If you are over sixty and want to try HT for the first time, find a doctor who will partner with you and closely monitor you, your symptoms, and your risk factors regularly if you decide to try it. But if you have been on HT since before age sixty, you don't need to stop taking it. "There's no stop date now," Dr. Kuhle told me.

BEYOND SEX HORMONES

Sex hormones aren't the only hormones coursing through our bodies. The endocrine system is command central for an extensive network of glands that produce the hormones needed to regulate not only sexual function, but also metabolism, growth, mood, and even aging itself. As we live longer, our body's production of many hormones decreases, and while others may stay the same, our body becomes less sensitive to them or less able to convert them to active forms. With hormones, though, it's not as simple as too much or too little—you really want those levels in their Goldilocks range of just right.

Here's a quick rundown of the non-reproductive hormone-related changes that happen with age. I share these with you because knowledge is power in ageless aging, and so many of these hormonal issues can be positively impacted with nutrition, movement, good sleep, effective stress management, and holistic healthcare.

Metabolic hormones

- **Insulin** modulates the amount of glucose in your bloodstream, which generally remains the same in terms of levels as we age. However, our insulin receptors become less sensitive, a condition known as *insulin resistance*. That means we tend to have higher blood glucose levels because insulin is less able to deliver its messages and move glucose out of the blood and into either muscle cells (for use) or fat cells (for storage). Minimizing refined sugars and eating more colorful produce will help keep glucose and insulin levels in a healthy range.

Adrenal gland hormones

- **Cortisol** is the stress hormone released by the cortex of the adrenal gland, and it tends to rise as we age, regardless of the stressors we are facing.[13] This increase is believed to negatively impact brain health, sleep, muscle mass, blood pressure, bone health, and abdominal circumference.[14] Women in menopause commonly have low cortisol during the day, making them feel tired, and high cortisol at night, which makes them worry. Steroid medications (such as prednisone) can elevate cortisol levels, as can excessive drinking and, of course, chronic or extreme stress. Our holistic recipe for ageless aging, including practicing relaxation and breathing (something we'll cover in the next chapter), eating a diet heavy in colorful anti-inflammatory plants, getting regular exercise, spending time in nature, and working with your circadian rhythm to get better sleep, can help bring cortisol levels down.
- **Dehydroepiandrosterone (DHEA)** is used by the body to produce both estrogen and testosterone, and levels of it naturally decline as we age. By the time you're seventy to eighty, your levels are only 10 to 20 percent of those of a twenty-year-old. Some small studies suggest that supplementing with DHEA can improve skin

firmness and reduce age spots, depression, and vaginal dryness.[15] But it's still controversial (Mayo Clinic gives it the red light—as in, avoid it—on their website). Supplementing carries a risk of tipping your estrogen and testosterone levels into the "too high" category (especially if you're also taking estradiol as part of your HT) and increasing insulin resistance. It may also increase the risk of hormone-sensitive cancers, is believed to lower levels of HDL (the good kind of cholesterol), and could exacerbate mood or psychiatric disorders. On top of that, DHEA supplements are not bioidentical. Full disclosure: I took DHEA when I had hip pain. I felt great, with more energy and vitality and less pain, but started getting heart palpitations, so I stopped taking it. While DHEA holds promise, it's not ready yet for prime time.

Growth hormones

- **Human growth hormone (HGH)**, which is very active when we're young, plays a role in protecting our muscles, bones, and organs and promoting the metabolism of fats. HGH naturally declines with age, which may seem like a bad thing, but it also has a good side, as lower levels of HGH and IGF-1 (another growth hormone I'll cover in just a minute) are associated with longevity. That's because the human body is either in grow-and-reproduce mode or in maintenance mode. And for longer life, we want to be in maintenance mode. So unless you are truly deficient in HGH, as diagnosed by a healthcare provider, you likely do *not* want to take HGH. Intermittent fasting, strength training, and regular sleep all appear to support healthy levels of HGH—yet another way that the holistic stone soup approach supports healthspan.

- **Insulin growth factor 1 (IGF-1)** is another growth hormone that we typically want to be at lower levels to promote healthy aging and longevity. As Dr. Valter Longo explained to me: "When IGF-1 gives the orders to grow, it's basically an order to your body to live life in the fast lane and not worry about maintenance." Also, there is an association between high IGF-1 levels and a higher incidence of cancer. Many things raise IGF-1 levels, including a high protein intake in those under sixty-five. That's why Longo recommends keeping protein intake moderate for those under sixty-five, as we covered in Chapter 5, and why after age sixty-five you can consume more protein because it can help you preserve muscle mass without the risk of increasing IGF-1. However, you do want some IGF-1, since it plays a role in the formation of new neurons and neuronal connections in the brain. Intermittent fasting helps keep those IGF-1 levels in a sweet spot, as they fall during your fasting period and then rise when you begin eating again.

Thyroid hormones

The thyroid gland controls metabolism and how your body uses energy. Dr. Seda Suvag, a board-certified endocrinologist at Memorial Regional Hospital in Hollywood, Florida, told me that the thyroid gland controls the rhythm of the body—from your heart rate to the cycles of the turnover of bone cells and cholesterol synthesis. The most common thyroid hormone imbalance in postmenopausal women is hypothyroidism, or a decreased level of thyroid hormone. This can be due to low levels of thyroid hormones or an autoimmune condition known as Hashimoto's thyroiditis, in which the immune system attacks the thyroid. In addition, more than 50 percent of adults age fifty and over have thyroid nodules, which can be assessed with a genetic test to see if they are cancerous (instead of being biopsied or removed outright, as was standard in the not-so-distant past).

Thyroid hormone imbalances manifest in different ways. For example, my close friend Kendra, a healthy and attractive seventy-one-year-old, started noticing dramatic changes in her hair. It became dry and brittle, breaking off regularly and falling out at an alarming rate. She went to a hair specialist, who took one look and said, "I see this a lot; you're probably hypothyroid." The specialist told her to get a blood test right away because there are safe medications that can adjust the levels of these hormones rather quickly. That's exactly what Kendra did, and it turns out she wasn't producing enough thyroid hormones, causing hair loss, weight gain, fatigue, and some forgetfulness. Her doctor prescribed Synthroid, and six months later, she looks and feels far better—and her hair is flourishing.

Hair loss, persistent fatigue, unexplained weight gain or loss, changing sensitivities to temperature, constipation, and changes in mood can all be related to thyroid issues. If you're experiencing any of these, let your primary care doctor know and ask them to check your thyroid levels, specifically your TSH, T4, and T3.

CUTTING-EDGE APPROACHES TO HORMONES

- **Menstrual mapping.** This urine-based test offered by ZRT Lab analyzes levels of estrogen, progesterone, and luteinizing hormone across the span of thirty days to offer a more dynamic portrait of your hormone levels than a onetime blood test. If you're perimenopausal, the test can help your HT doctor see whether giving you some low levels of estrogen and/or progesterone might be able to smooth out the curves in your hormonal roller coaster. (If you're postmenopausal, you don't need this test.) Dr. Gersh told me that she uses menstrual mapping regularly in her practice to identify women who are still cycling but who could benefit from what she called "giving a little cushion" of HT to ease their perimenopausal symptoms. You need a healthcare provider to order the test for you—refer them to zrtlabs.com.

- **Mirena IUD instead of progesterone for HT.** You don't necessarily have to take progesterone with your bioidentical estrogen in order to minimize the risk of endometrial cancer—you could use Mirena to serve the same function. Mirena was developed as a form of birth control, so using it to deliver progesterone is an off-label usage. The hormone the IUD secretes at very low levels over time—levonorgestrel, which is the same active ingredient in the Plan B morning-after pill—also thins the uterine lining and protects against the risk of endometrial cancer in women who are at or beyond the end of their reproductive years. Dr. Kuhle told me, "If I see a patient who does not want to take progesterone for any reason—they aren't great at remembering to take it, for example—I suggest the Mirena. I have given them to women in their seventies. They're good for five to seven years and then all you do is put your estradiol patch on." Kate also has a friend who used Mirena as birth control and then had it removed when she was going through menopause, per her doctor's orders—and then her menopause symptoms kicked into high gear. (She's been trying to find a doctor who will prescribe her a new one ever since.) That's the hitch—many OB/GYNs won't prescribe Mirena to women fifty and over. Again, you need to find a doctor certified in menopausal medicine. If your insurance won't cover it, the out-of-pocket cost is $1,100 at the time of this writing.

- **Suppositories for vaginal health.** Imvexxy is an estradiol suppository (imvexxy.com) that you insert directly into the vagina to counteract the vaginal dryness, burning, itching, and atrophy that often occur with menopause and can lead to painful sex and frequent urinary infections. Delivering estrogen straight to the vagina can help your vaginal and vulvar tissues regenerate themselves and can be a good option if your primary symptoms are painful sex or frequent urinary infections and for some reason you don't want to take a bigger dose of estradiol via patch or pill. You do need a prescription, and your doctor can help determine the dosage.

Another option is a hyaluronic acid (HA) suppository. Revaree is one such option that is hormone-free and available without a prescription. HA is a molecule your body produces naturally that is used in many facial products because it can retain up to a thousand times its weight in moisture, helping your cells stay strong and hydrated. "We're putting it on our face—why not on all mucous membranes?" Dr. Ramonas said. Either suppository option can be a good first approach to improving vaginal integrity and health—and a less invasive and expensive alternative to some of the laser vaginal rejuvenation treatments offered by some gynecologists and plastic surgeons.

HORMONE HEALTH: WHERE TO BEGIN

If you do one thing: Get a bone density test

A bone density scan (DEXA scan) will allow you to see if your bones are being compromised by lack of estrogen/progesterone. Although the U.S. Preventive Services Task Force does not recommend getting a DEXA scan until you are sixty-five, other organizations such as the Bone Health and Osteoporosis Foundation suggest getting one if you are fifty or older and have a risk of fracture (such as a parent who has had broken a hip).

Dr. Kuhle told me that having osteopenia is an important consideration for going on HT, as it can prevent the development of full-blown osteoporosis. "We commonly see women who went through menopause like a year or two before, and they have not been on hormone therapy, and they are very surprised that they have lost some bone already." A DEXA scan is how you find out if you have low bone density—or not.

A DEXA scan is a quick, painless procedure that uses very low-dose radiation to measure the density of your bones at specific places— typically the pelvis, the top of the femur, and your lower spine.

If you are found to have osteopenia or osteoporosis, you'll likely be referred to an endocrinologist, not an orthopedic doctor—that's how closely bone health is tied to hormonal balance. "Bone is an endocrine organ," Dr. Gersh explained. "Bone itself makes hormones, and the hormones that bones make help control glucose regulation and cognition. So women with less bone will tend to have less cognitive ability and be more likely to have diabetes and insulin resistance."

If you're a beginner: Find a qualified doctor certified in menopause medicine

I didn't know it before doing research for this book, but the Menopause Society (MS) certifies doctors in menopausal medicine. You can do a search at portal.menopause.org to find a doctor near you. You may need a referral from your primary care doctor or OB/GYN (this is what Kate needed to get an appointment with the MS-certified doctor in her area, and she had to have her OB/GYN's office actually fax the referral to the menopause clinic—even in this digital age), and you may need to place your name on a wait list. Still, it is worth it to find a doctor educated about menopause.

Once you find a doctor, go in with your Menopause Rating Scale, notes on any other symptoms that might be related to peri- or post-menopause, and information on your family health history that can highlight your individual risks. Ask the doctor, "What is your knowledge or interest in hormone therapy? Are you committed to using bioidentical hormones? How long do you feel women should be on it if their symptoms and clinical history suggest that they would benefit from it?" Listen to their answers with your ears, your mind, and your gut. "If you feel the doctor pooh-poohs your concerns or doesn't seem to have a good grasp of the latest findings on MHT, you need to find somebody else," Dr. Kuhle advised.

If you want to take your hormonal investigations to the next level: Understand the hidden link between low thyroid levels, elevated cholesterol levels, and the risk of heart disease

I regularly get blood tests to check cholesterol levels (which run high in my family), thyroid levels, and everything in between. A few years ago, my test results revealed a few levels that were out of whack, including elevated LDL and low thyroid. My doctor immediately put me on a medication called Synthroid and let me know that it would not only help improve my thyroid gland's functioning, but lower my cholesterol levels and risk of heart disease as well. Recognize that there is a holistic relationship between our different hormone levels and potential health risk factors.

— ◆ —

AGELESS AGING HACKS
TO HELP HORMONES HELP YOU

Eat edamame and other (organic) soy products

Soybeans, in addition to being a good source of protein and fiber, are rich in isoflavones—one of several compounds known as phytoestrogens, which are structurally and functionally very similar to human estrogen. Once you are perimenopausal or postmenopausal, consuming soy products can help naturally boost your estrogen levels. Ideally, you'd eat organic soy that has been fermented—such as tempeh, miso, and natto—because fermentation is beneficial for your microbiome and can make the nutrients in soy even more bioavailable. (Conventional soybeans tend to be genetically modified, so organic soy is best.) One caveat: If you or a close female relative has had a hormone-sensitive cancer, such as breast, uterine, or ovarian cancer, consult with a registered dietitian, functional medicine doctor, or naturopathic doctor who has been trained in nutrition to determine if this is a healthy and safe choice for you.

If you are a breast cancer survivor and need to cope with menopausal symptoms

Certain antidepressant and antianxiety medications, at lower doses, can be a great alternative. For example, Brisdelle and Paxil (both brand names for paroxetine) have FDA approval for reducing the vasomotor symptoms of perimenopause and menopause, such as hot flashes and night sweats, although many docs prescribe other SSRIs, such as Celexa (citalopram) and Lexapro (escitalopram), and SNRIs, such as Effexor (venlafaxine) and Pristiq (desvenlafaxine), off-label to achieve the same effects. One important note: paroxetine can interfere with the breast cancer treatment drug tamoxifen, so if you need that medication, you likely want to avoid Brisdelle and Paxil. Switching to an SNRI such as Effexor may be a better fit and equally effective. As always, check with your doctor.

If you want to slow the process of collagen loss in your skin

Estrogen stimulates collagen production in our skin cells. That means that as we age and our estrogen levels decline, collagen levels drop, too, creating changes in our skin. While skin care is not a primary reason to start taking hormones, HT can help protect your skin. You also can stimulate collagen production in other ways. Skincare products with the right ingredients, such as vitamin C, hyaluronic acid, and retinols, can be helpful. (Consistent use of these products is key.) Eating adequate amounts of lean proteins that contain amino acids critical for collagen synthesis is also beneficial. Marine collagen is a great supplement for firmer skin. And eliminating most sugar is essential, since it can break down the collagen in your skin. Of course, the holistic recipe for ageless aging includes many of these and other suggestions that help stimulate collagen growth in our skin, such as a great night's sleep, avoiding stress, and regular exercise.

If you take an SSRI and experience low libido or an inability to have an orgasm

Switching to a different antidepressant may restore your sex drive. While depression itself can zap libido in as many as 50 percent of people who suffer from it, sometimes the decline in sex drive is due to the medication itself, particularly Brisdelle (paroxetine), Celexa (citalopram), Lexapro (escitalopram), Luvox (fluvoxamine), Paxil (paroxetine), Prozac (fluoxetine), Trintellix (vortioxetine), and Zoloft (sertraline). A known side effect of SSRIs is a lowered interest in sex, reduced arousal, and impaired ability to have an orgasm, and this side effect becomes more common with age. If this is you, talk to your doctor about switching to Remeron (mirtazapine) or Wellbutrin (bupropion), which are antidepressants that don't have sexual side effects. Having that connection and release is well worth it!

If you are still pre- or perimenopausal and experiencing low sex drive that has come out of nowhere

First talk to your primary care doctor about screening you for depression, as low libido can be a side effect. And if that's not the root, consider Addyi (flibanserin), which is a little pink pill, or Vyleesi (bremelanotide), which is an easy-to-self-administer injection, to help raise your sex drive. We hear a lot about Viagra and Cialis for men, but less about the prescription drugs that help women with low sex drive. Addyi and Vyleesi are those drugs. Compounded testosterone may also help.

If you are postmenopausal and experiencing painful sex

In addition to the suppositories I covered earlier in this chapter, you can try intravaginal DHEA. The loss of estrogen can cause the tissues in your vagina to thin. While some docs will prescribe vaginal estrogen to treat painful sex, administering DHEA to the site can also be helpful (and has no limitations on how long you can use it, unlike typical vaginal estrogens—although it's important to note that you don't need to use both; it's either vaginal estrogen or vaginal DHEA). Intrarosa is a vaginal insert delivering DHEA directly to the vagina to help ease painful sex. Your body will convert the DHEA to estrogen. Again, talk to your doctor, especially if you have or have had breast cancer or have a family history of the disease.

9

❖

YOUR BEAUTIFUL MIND

Now that you've experimented with some of the essential ingredients related to your body, it's time to zero in on your mind and spirit. Cultivating better brain health—and, just as importantly, emotional health and a positive attitude—is like fairy dust sprinkled on top of all those other lifestyle habits to animate and vitalize your life. There's a lot of scientific data that points to the holistic connection between our thoughts, our attitudes, our brain health, and our overall healthspan and lifespan. The ageless aging holistic recipe really comes into full focus when it comes to our beautiful minds.

In every research study Age Wave has conducted in recent years—even during the height of the COVID lockdowns—the number-one health fear for women fifty and over has been Alzheimer's disease and cognitive decline. While heart disease is the number-one killer of women, we are terrified that our bodies might outlive our brains.

The truth is, we're right to be worried. One-third of all people eighty-five and older have some form of dementia, and two-thirds of all people with Alzheimer's disease are women. It's not just because we live longer than men. Although we're not completely sure why, we do know the loss of estrogen and progesterone due to menopause is a contributor (another reason to consider MHT). Dr. Lisa Mosconi, director of the Alzheimer's Prevention Clinic and the Women's Brain

Initiative at Weill Cornell Medicine, writes in her book *The XX Brain*, "Menopause doesn't 'cause' Alzheimer's. Menopause is more like a trigger in which the superpower of estrogen and its companion hormones is revoked."

OLD-SCHOOL THINKING ABOUT
DEMENTIA IS OUT OF DATE

Until recently, the pervasive thinking around dementia was that there wasn't much you could do to change the hand genetics dealt you. I'm happy to share the great news that today we know the genetic connection to Alzheimer's is overstated. "Fewer than four percent of Alzheimer's patients have a genetic component to their disease," Dr. Andrea Pfeifer, a medical researcher as well as co-founder of AC Immune, a Swiss biopharmaceutical company focused on developing treatments for Alzheimer's disease, told me.

On top of that, there have been woefully few medications approved for treatment or prevention of dementia. Several drugs have shown a limited impact, slowing the symptoms for a short while, but they are largely ineffective and have many side effects. That only recently began to change when two drugs received FDA approval in 2021 and 2023—aducanumab (Aduhelm) and lecanemab (Leqembi)—with a third about to gain FDA approval, donanemab. The great news about these medications is that they are the first treatments that have been shown to reduce the progression of the brain plaques that are a hallmark of the disease. The bad news is that even the FDA and the Alzheimer's Association admit these treatments are only "reasonably likely to lead to a reduction in clinical decline due to Alzheimer's disease." Oh, and the side effects include the risk of brain bleeds, sometimes referred to as brain tattoos, that require MRIs to assess.

Ann Seclow, a friend and psychotherapist who has the APOE4 gene that increases the risk of Alzheimer's and has been identified as already having plaques in her brain, was screened for the clinical trial of lecanemab. She told me that, after much probing, she learned that the side effects are far riskier for women with the APOE4 gene than for men, which is not mentioned in the literature. She told me she had to "pull that fact out with lots of deep questioning."

Still, these are first-generation drugs—their mere existence is a triumph. As Lisa Genova, a neuroscientist and author of the novel *Still Alice* (the basis for an Academy Award–winning film), told me, "If we look at cancer or HIV and AIDS, the first drugs to market weren't a home run. It was version 1.0." She went on to say, "I'm very much encouraged and hopeful about the drugs that will follow in version 2.0, 3.0. I think they will have fewer side effects and be less invasive—maybe it will be a patch or a nasal spray." She also explained that, similar to how treatments for HIV developed over time, there will likely be a cocktail of drugs. In fact, researchers are currently working on drugs that target tau tangles (another marker of Alzheimer's) and neuroinflammation. And there are several vaccines in the works as well.

Most importantly, "there is a massive cultural shift taking place, both for general practice doctors and the general public," Genova explained. It's becoming more widely known that we do have agency over the health of our brains—we can take steps that are likely to delay or prevent Alzheimer's and other cognitive decline through our own actions. In fact, some doctors are beginning to say, "In addition to the drug we can offer you, we want you to eat healthier, exercise, sleep, and manage your stress."

Some doctors already are going even further and utilizing cutting-edge diagnostic tools to determine a woman's risk of Alzheimer's disease and other cognitive disorders. In her book *The XX Brain*, Lisa Mosconi recommends getting either a CT scan, an MRI, or—if possible—even a PET scan of your brain. Since dementia begins to develop decades before there are symptoms, these early screeners could identify plaques, tangles, and other changes in brain tissue, as well as up the odds of catching a brain tumor or aneurysm early, when it is much more treatable. Chances are, you'll have to advocate for these diagnostic tools. And PET scans are, at the time of this writing, typically only available to cancer patients or participants in clinical research trials. But, Mosconi writes, "I look forward to the day when we will routinely peek inside a woman's head and use *her* brain as our guide to provide the best recommendations specific to optimizing *her* health . . . much in the same way a current female's middle-age healthcare routine includes mammograms."

My friend Meryl Comer, a fellow co-founder of Women Against Alzheimer's, a board member of Us Against Alzheimer's, a prominent Alzheimer's advocate, and bestselling author who spent more than two decades being a caregiver for her husband and her mother, who both suffered from Alzheimer's, sums it up perfectly: "We women must do more to keep our brains healthy until the science catches up."

What's Normal Cognitive Aging, and What's a Warning Sign?

The fear of getting dementia can torment you. I know this fear firsthand since my mother died with Alzheimer's disease, and it haunts me. I do everything in my power to prevent and delay the disease. I also know that fear spikes whenever you find yourself having small lapses in memory. Lisa Genova told me that after every speech she gives, women approach her in the ladies' room and say something like, "I'm always forgetting people's names," or "I walk into a room, and I don't know why I'm there. Does this mean I'm getting Alzheimer's? Do I already have it?"

"There's this misconception that memory is supposed to be perfect. So we take any signs of cognitive decline as abnormal," she told me. "If you park your car in the parking garage, go shopping, and when you come back out you go, 'Oh my God, I can't remember where I parked my car!' that is normal." In order to remember something, you need to pay attention, so if you were texting on your way into the store or already thinking about what you were going to buy, you simply didn't lay that memory down. This same thing happens when you set your keys or phone down—you can't remember where you put them because you were distracted when you set them down. "You haven't actually forgotten anything—you never made the memory in the first place," Genova explained. "What's worrisome is if you park the car, go into the mall, and then don't remember how you got there. Or if you are standing in front of your car, but you don't recognize it as yours."

Another thing that's normal, Genova tells me, is taking longer to remember words or recover your train of thought. "Our processing speeds slow down as we age. It feels like that little rainbow circle spinning on your computer," she explained. The electrochemical signals in your brain are not as fast as they used to be. So when you struggle to remember someone's name, don't beat yourself up. Instead, go look it up. "By looking it up instead of suffering, you're actually freeing up your brain to do other things that are useful," Genova explained.

That said, there are ways to train your brain to function better. They're likely not the things you think. Forget crosswords, Wordle, and Sudoku. They won't cut it. Neither will many of the cognitive training apps and digital programs. "You're going to get really good at those games by practicing them, but that doesn't help you better remember last year's vacation or your memories from college, or what you have to pick up at the grocery store later," Genova told me.

Here are six things you can do that *will* help expand your cognitive resilience.

- **Figure things out for yourself.** When your dishwasher breaks or your iPad doesn't work, don't just call a repair person or ask your partner or child to fix it. Look up how to fix the problem online and do it yourself. You'll be building self-reliance and encouraging new neuronal connections.
- **Be a lifelong learner.** You're never too old to learn something new and be a beginner. New learning helps you stay curious, stimulates your brain, and fosters neuroplasticity.
- **Revisit, repeat, again and again.** Lisa Genova told me, "If you want to hold on to new learnings, you need to revisit the information again and again." Keep practicing it so those new associations and skills are laid down more permanently.

> - **Do the math.** When you go out to dinner, calculate the tip in your head, or if you're splitting the bill with friends, do the division without a calculator. When you're balancing your checkbook, calculate the numbers first in your head, then check them with a calculator.
> - **Seek out the new and novel.** Novelty is your brain's friend. For example, explore new-to-you cuisines, both in eating and in cooking, to build cognitive muscle. Likewise, find new routes to drive or walk to get where you need to go without relying on GPS.

YOUR TO-DO LIST TO REDUCE RISK
OF COGNITIVE DECLINE

For too long, the medical establishment believed that it is not possible to prevent or delay cognitive decline. Not anymore. Scientific data published in 2017 in *The Lancet,* one of the oldest and most respected medical journals, provided a significant body of evidence that addressing ten risk factors can reduce the risk of developing dementia by as much as 40 percent.[1] Then, in 2020, *The Lancet* updated that report to include two new risk factors.[2] You can't help but assume researchers will continue to find evidence of more lifestyle changes to increase brainspan. As the authors of the guidelines wrote, "It is never too early and never too late in the life course for dementia prevention."

Let's look at those risk factors, as well as what you can do to mitigate them and improve your brainspan.

- **Stimulate your brain by learning new things.** As I mentioned above, being a lifelong learner has many benefits. Education in early life (before the age of forty-five) builds cognitive reserve, increasing your brain's capacity and resilience, making you less vulnerable to dementia. One theory as to why women who are currently in their seventies, eighties, and nineties have such a higher risk of developing dementia than men is that they typically received less education than men decades ago. But why stop learning as we live longer? Continuing to learn and study new things once you're forty-five and older helps maintain brainspan.

- **Minimize diabetes risk.** If you have type 2 diabetes or are prediabetic, it's time to take action—buy a glucose monitor, and eat fewer refined carbs and more colorful vegetables as well as healthy fats, as I outlined in Chapter 5—and get those fasting glucose and insulin levels into a healthy range.

- **Treat high blood pressure.** Stiff blood vessels mean higher blood pressure and restricted blood flow, including to the brain. New York cardiologist Dr. Suzanne Steinbaum told me that if your doctor suggests you lower your blood pressure with medication, it doesn't mean you failed. It means you have an opportunity to do better for both your heart and your brain.

- **Protect your hearing.** Hearing stimulates the brain, which means impaired hearing can cause the brain to atrophy. If needed, wearing a hearing aid mitigates the cognitive risk of hearing loss. Get checked by an audiologist (especially if your partner, family, or friends tell you that your hearing is declining) and if they prescribe hearing aids—or you've previously been fitted for hearing aids—wear them! At this writing, Harvard scientists have developed a potentially groundbreaking solution to hearing loss in the form of molecules that can regenerate hair cells in the ear, improving hearing.[3] Hopefully, this will be in clinical trials and approved and available sometime soon.

- **Stop smoking.** Smoking is terrible for your lungs, brutal on your bones, and bad for your brain. If you are reading this book, you clearly care about taking care of yourself. Smoking works directly against that desire—even if you only smoke socially or occasionally. Anecdotally, I hear that hypnotism can be helpful for quitting. Minimizing your exposure to secondhand smoke is also important.

- **Manage your weight.** No judgment here, but true obesity—as opposed to being overweight according to clinical definitions—has been associated with dementia risk by dozens of studies. Weight loss of only 4.4 pounds has been tied to significant improvements in memory and attention among study participants with a mean age of fifty.[4]

- **Treat your depression.** Depression is sometimes a symptom of early cognitive decline. Remember the U-curve of happiness we covered in Chapter 2, which describes how happiness tends to bottom out in the forties and then to start rising in the fifties? If you don't feel yourself climbing the upward side of the happiness curve, seek out therapy and, if needed, medication and activities that help reduce depression symptoms.

- **Exercise, exercise, exercise.** Nearly every expert I interviewed for this book named exercise as the number-one thing they do to protect their healthspan and particularly their brainspan. It is as protective for your brain as it is for your heart, increasing blood flow and delivering nutrients into all cells, including those in your brain, which results in more energy generation. It also produces molecules known as exerkines—including BDNF—that boost neurogenesis (the formation of new neurons) and neuroplasticity.

- **Connect with others.** Loneliness is a proven risk factor for dementia, likely because social interaction enhances cognitive reserve. Being around other people, especially interesting and open-minded people, can also help you see things more positively, help you get things off your chest, offer new perspectives, and encourage you to do more of the things that are good for you. We'll cover this in depth in the next chapter.

- **Cut back on alcohol.** While a glass of red wine can be a welcome stress reliever and a source of antioxidants, the bottom line is that alcohol is a neurotoxin. We've known for centuries that heavy drinking is a cognitive risk. Now we understand that even moderate drinking can be, too. As Ann Seclow told me, "I'm trying to build brain cells, not kill them, so I seldom drink anymore." Stick to the guideline of no more than one drink per day (that means five ounces of wine, twelve ounces of beer, or one ounce of hard liquor).

- **Protect your head.** Traumatic brain injury is a clear risk factor for dementia. Just as you wear a seatbelt in the car, wear your helmet any time you are on a bike, skis, skates, skateboard, or scooter. Consider installing a handrail on outdoor stairs, removing or replacing slippery throw rugs, and improving lighting in dark areas where it might be easy to misstep.

- **Minimize indoor air pollution.** Indoor air can be even more polluted than outdoor air, and pollutants can be harmful to your brain. Open your windows, even when it's cold or hot outside. Consider an air filter for your home—at least in your bedroom, where your brain repairs and refreshes itself overnight. And skip synthetic home fragrances, whether they are plug-ins, sprays, or candles, as synthetic fragrance is generally toxic.

- **Cut out ultra-processed foods.** Although this isn't yet included on *The Lancet*'s list of modifiable risk factors for dementia, I'm sure it will be in a future update. Research published in 2022 followed nearly eleven thousand Brazilian adults for over a decade and revealed a connection between eating ultra-processed foods—such as chips, sodas, hot dogs, chicken nuggets, and other packaged foods—and an accelerated decline in cognitive functioning.[5] The good news is that the cognitive risk was mitigated when people mostly ate a healthy, Mediterranean diet rich in whole foods.

MORE TO-DOS TO SAFEGUARD YOUR BRAINSPAN

The brain is mysterious and still not fully understood by science. "There's a special kind of taboo about anything that's happening from the neck up," Lisa Genova explained to me. "It's a universe inside our head—literally billions of neurons with ten thousand connections each. It's an unfathomable amount of connectivity and data and processing all within the three pounds inside our closed skull."

We know the brain influences every part of the body and that there are additional influences on brain health beyond those that have been included on *The Lancet*'s list. While it may seem overwhelming that there are so many factors that contribute to brain health, the flip side is there are so many levers we can pull to protect and even improve our brainspans, including:

- **Hormones.** Between premenopause and postmenopause, the average woman's brain scans show a stark decline in brain activity. That's because estrogen is neuroprotective, guarding our neurons from infection and promoting neuroplasticity. It also promotes blood flow to the brain and plays a key role in the function of specific regions associated with memory, attention, and planning.[6] It's yet another reason to talk to your doctor to see if MHT is a fit for you.

- **Sleep.** As described in Chapter 6, sleep is when the brain takes out its own trash via the glymphatic system, as well as consolidates memories. The average quality and quantity of your sleep matters, and as I've described, there are many strategies to improve your sleep.

- **Stress.** Stress is complicated, necessary, and not always bad for you. But when you respond to situations by feeling anxious or overly threatened, that's negative stress or *distress*. Distress is bad, contributing to inflammation, accelerating biological aging, and triggering "inflammaging," the deterioration of the immune system. Some of this is because stress triggers the formation of senescent cells, those pro-inflammatory zombie cells we covered in Chapter 1, and shortens telomeres, the protective caps at the end of each chromosome that can prevent chromosome degradation and premature aging. This equates directly to more inflammation, which means shorter brainspans, healthspans, and lifespans. When distress becomes chronic, "it breaks the shutoff valve in your brain that controls the release of cortisol and adrenaline, which is super bad for our brains," Genova explained to me. When we get locked into the stress response, "it makes it very difficult for us to retrieve information we know, to lay down new memories, and probably puts us at greater risk for Alzheimer's."

On the other hand, positive stress, or what is called *eustress*, can be good for you. Experiences that are intense but pleasurable, such as getting a promotion, finishing a project with a tight deadline, or meeting a new grandchild for the first time, are examples of positive stress. In short, eustress is a key to survival and long life, while distress can lead to serious health risks.

Mindfulness training—there are many different forms—is a great technique for coping with and becoming more resilient to distress. It can literally *change your brain*. For instance, studies of people who have meditated for many years have shown that the long-term meditators had more cortical thickness, which protects against normal age-related brain thinning that's linked to dementia. A seminal Harvard study found that participants in an eight-week mindfulness-based stress reduction class, which met once a week, supplemented by audio recordings that students could follow at home, increased the density of gray matter in the hippocampus—the brain region involved in learning and memory—and in other parts of the brain that are associated with self-awareness, compassion, and introspection.[7] Meditation also leads to greater mental clarity and less anxiety.

Like the positivity effect, reframing is another valuable tool for managing stress. It's a learned skill that's all about looking at a situation through a more positive lens. While many stressors are beyond our control, it is within our control to pick and choose what we get stressed by. "I will not allow myself to get stressed over something stupid that happened, because it's not worth the energy," Carolee Lee, an entrepreneur who is founder and CEO of WHAM (Women's Health Access Matters), told me. She suggested asking yourself questions that redirect your focus, such as: *What can I fix? How could I make someone happy? How could I feel like I've made the world a better place? What am I grateful for?*

- **Gut health.** Earlier, we talked about the bacteria in your gut known as the microbiome and the large role it plays in brain health. In fact, the gut is known as the second brain. Beneficial bacteria manufacture neurotransmitters and nutrients that help prevent infection. This last part is important because many bacteria and viruses and their byproducts are linked to dementia, including *Porphyromonas gingivalis*, which is responsible for gum disease; the herpes virus, responsible for cold sores, genital sores, and shingles; and the protein alpha-synuclein, which is shed by bad gut bacteria and has been linked to Parkinson's. "If your microbiome is in a good place, you can make antibodies to fight these viruses and to break up the amyloid plaques," Pfeifer explained to me. She told me that probiotics are the only supplement she takes. Besides taking probiotics, you can eat fermented foods and prioritize high-fiber foods to strengthen your population of good gut bacteria. In addition, cutting down on sugar deprives the bad bacteria of their favorite food source and helps the good bacteria crowd out the bad.

  Another benefit of better gut health is that it is directly linked to positive emotions, such as happiness, as well as to better emotional coping skills.[8]

- **Inflammation.** This buzzword is all about a healthy immune response gone wrong, leading to the degradation of healthy tissues. Not surprisingly, inflammation can happen in the brain. Current thinking is that neuroinflammation increases the production of amyloid protein, which contributes to plaques, while simultaneously reducing the glymphatic system's ability to clear amyloid out of the brain. In addition, neuroinflammation can target and kill healthy neurons. Eating the rainbow, as we discussed in Chapter 5, becomes even more important when you know that the antioxidants that make fruits and vegetables colorful also help reduce inflammation throughout the body. So does getting plenty of omega-3 fatty acids, whether through wild fatty fish such as salmon or through supplements, which I discuss later in this chapter.

Supplements for Stress and Brain Health

There are certain nutrients that are extra-important for brain health, and herbs that can help your body better handle stress. While most doctors will tell you to get your nutrients from food instead of supplements, who has a perfect diet? The brain-supportive supplements listed below are the basics; I've also included some supplements that can help counteract the negative effects of stress.

My one caveat is that the world of supplements can be very confusing, even misleading, as the supplement industry is not regulated by the FDA. That means your supplement may not contain what the label says it does, or it may have been manufactured in such a way that toxins get introduced into the product. I suggest working with a practitioner such as your primary care doctor, a nutritionist or registered dietitian, or a functional medicine doctor who can test your nutrient levels, help you determine which supplements you truly need, and recommend brands they trust to offer products that are readily bioavailable. If that's not an option, there are some home tests available, but do your research on supplement companies. Some companies jump through hoops to purify and test their products and will provide information on their website about where they source their ingredients and what kinds of testing they put their products through. Taking these steps makes their manufacturing process lengthier and more expensive, and they'll want you to know about it.

Brain Health Supplements

Probiotics. Andrea Pfeifer told me about the power of probiotics to support your microbiome *and* your brain health. Look for supplements that offer at least 10 billion colony-forming units (CFU), combined, of at least three different strains of bacteria. When you finish a bottle of one probiotic, purchase a different one next, as a variety of bacterial strains helps promote a thriving microbiome.

B complex. The family of B vitamins helps boost the production of neurotransmitters, and it's very common for women fifty and over to be deficient in them. One particular B vitamin, B12, is primarily found in animal-derived foods, so if you're a vegetarian or a vegan, you either need to prioritize eating nutritional yeast, the one plant-based source, or talk with your doctor about taking it in supplement form. There are a lot of retail operations that offer B vitamins in an infusion or a shot, supposedly making it far more bioavailable. Do not take B vitamins with vitamin C; vitamin C will not allow the B vitamins to be absorbed.

Omega-3s. Considered a nootropic, or brain enhancer, higher levels of these essential fatty acids have been associated with more gray matter in the hippocampus, lower anxiety, and the presence of fewer amyloid plaques.[9] Look for a purified brand, as most fish are contaminated with mercury.

Nootropics. These include a wide variety of substances that are touted as brain enhancers or "smart drugs" and that claim to improve memory, focus, creativity, and motivation. They vary from drugs such as Adderall to a wide range of supplements and even caffeine. You've probably seen print or television ads for some of these supplements that promise to boost cognitive performance; the options are too vast to evaluate for the mission of this book. Many doctors and longevity experts market their own blends of nootropics. Yet the body of evidence to support their efficacy and safety often doesn't exist. The nootropic compounds that show the most promise are L-theanine, a component found in green tea (and which also can help you sleep better, as I covered in Chapter 6); CDP-choline or citicoline, a naturally occurring molecule; creatine monohydrate, a dietary supplement that increases the production of the energy molecule ATP; and *Bacopa monnieri*, an herb used in traditional Indian medicine to promote the formation of new neuronal networks.[10]

Stress Supplements

Gamma-aminobutyric acid (GABA). This amino acid is an inhibitory neurotransmitter that, in supplement form, can quiet the brain, helping with stress and sleep. While scientific evidence of its effectiveness is mixed, research suggests that it requires continual use, at least a week, in order for noticeable changes to occur. I take it and love the calming effect it has on my racing mind when I wake up in the middle of the night.

Lemon balm. This herb is also considered to be a calming agent that doesn't put you to sleep, meaning you can take it any time of day. I take lemon balm, following the package instructions, if I'm feeling really anxious, and it does the trick. It also has a positive impact on your brain.

Ashwagandha and other adaptogens. Used in Ayurveda and traditional Chinese medicine for centuries, ashwagandha is an herbal adaptogen, which means it brings you back into balance—if you are overamped, it can lower your cortisol levels, and if you are worn out, it can raise them. It is a nerve tonic. A 2019 double-blind, randomized, controlled study found that people who took an ashwagandha supplement twice daily for eight weeks reported significantly lower stress levels than those who took a placebo.[11] Other adaptogenic herbs include American ginseng, Asian ginseng, eleuthero, and rhodiola.

THE HIDDEN MINDSET SUPERPOWER

Study after study points to the fact that keeping your thoughts focused on more positive outcomes may be a key to matching brainspan, healthspan, and lifespan. This is true even after accounting for lifestyle factors like smoking, excessive alcohol use, and poor nutrition. Don't forget Dr. Becca Levy's research, discussed in Chapter 1, which showed that people with a heightened genetic risk for dementia (because they have the APOE4 gene) who had a positive view of aging essentially erased their greater risk of developing dementia. Dr. Levy described cultivating a more positive mindset as "addressing the enemy from within."[12]

It's important to note that facing a problem head-on needn't be all work—nor should it be. "If you just try to reduce all your risk factors, but you feel unhappy for the last twenty years of your life, or stressed about all the things you could be doing, it's completely missing the point," Gaël Chételat, PhD, a leading Alzheimer's researcher, explained. Focusing on the fun and empowerment you feel while doing the things that can extend your healthspan is a vital part of the recipe, as is savoring how much better they make you feel. A way to foster those good feelings is to focus on the activities that help you feel connected to others and give you a sense of purpose and meaning—which is exactly what we'll cover in the next chapter.

CUTTING-EDGE APPROACHES TO BRAIN HEALTH

- **Preventive neurology.** What should already exist but doesn't is the ability to see a neurologist when you are cognitively fine to develop a preventive neurologic plan for your future. You may have to educate yourself and then push the healthcare system to meet you where the science is. Ann Seclow told me this from her firsthand experience when being assessed for the lecanemab clinical trial: "Even the neurologists at UCSF, who were stellar doctors, say they're not ready to work with patients to develop a preventive plan for Alzheimer's. The insurance codes for this type of preventive work don't even exist yet. So, I had to go outside the system to find a preventive neurologist." Not surprisingly, this doctor is a woman, and she is open to learning and helping Ann set up baselines and biomarkers and work with the latest research in the field. "It's possible to work with a healthcare provider on extending your brainspan," Ann says, "but it's going to take a little more work because the system's not set up for it."

- **New diagnostic blood test for Alzheimer's disease.** Until recently, the diagnostics for Alzheimer's disease have required either a postmortem autopsy or a PET imaging scan to assess the level of amyloid plaques and tau tangles in the brain. (While both are considered a hallmark of Alzheimer's disease, they are not a smoking gun—some Alzheimer's patients have very few plaques and tangles, while some cognitively healthy people are found to have a significant amount of them. Nonetheless, they are an important biomarker for brain health.) Now there is a long-awaited blood test that assesses the level of amyloid or tau in your bloodstream and even in your brain. These tests are available from LabCorp (labcorp.com). You will need a doctor to help you better assess the results; start with your primary care physician and ask for a referral to a specialist if you still would like more information on what your results mean.

- **Microdosing.** Although the practice is illegal in most states, it seems I can hardly talk to anyone, whether they are friends of my adult children or my own friends and colleagues, without the topic of microdosing coming up. Microdosing means taking a small amount of psychedelics—typically psilocybin (the psychoactive compound in magic mushrooms), or LSD—so small that your ability to function at work and tend to your daily responsibilities isn't impaired. In fact, it may improve your performance. Anecdotally, the word about microdosing is that it gives a subtle but noticeable uptick in mood, energy, and focus without the actual high. Using psychedelic drugs to treat mental and cognitive health was popularized by Michael Pollan's 2019 book *How to Change Your Mind.* Now, many people have started experimenting themselves—influenced by widespread stories of Silicon Valley executives and other biohackers espousing the benefits of psychedelics. What does this mean for the rest of us? Well, these drugs are still illegal in most places, though the FDA has granted psychedelics "breakthrough therapy" status, meaning they are legal for scientific research. So far, the science around whether microdosing is effective at improving mood, reducing symptoms of depression, and improving performance on cognitive tests is limited and inconclusive.[13] Microdoses of LSD have been shown to increase BDNF in a very small group of healthy humans, suggesting it does increase neuroplasticity. Some research suggests that long-term microdosing could negatively impact your heart, though most negative reports involve accidentally taking too much and experiencing more psychedelic effects than desired.[14]

- **Vagus nerve stimulation.** The vagus nerve, which I mentioned earlier in terms of sleep, is the primary nerve of the parasympathetic nervous system. In Latin, *vagus* means "wanderer," and this tenth cranial nerve travels from the brainstem, through the face and neck, through the heart and lungs, and all the way to the gut. Many refer to it as the "gut-brain superhighway" because it is thought to be the prime mode of communication between the brain and the organs of digestion. While there's still a lot we don't yet understand about the vagus nerve, we do know that it is involved in how your body registers safety and reacts to stress. Recent research has pointed to the potential benefits of using a noninvasive electrical device to stimulate the vagus nerve in order to treat, among other things, stress and depression as well as to lower chronic inflammation.[15] There are already FDA-approved devices on the market designed to stimulate the vagus nerve through electrical impulses, such as the Pulsetto, Apollo Wearable, Sensate, and Nurosym, which can range from $200 to $700, and I'm sure there will be many more to come. Other methods to stimulate the vagus nerve that haven't yet been studied to the extent that FDA-approved devices have include massage or cold exposure (especially on your neck), meditation, laughing, singing, and deep breathing—many of the things we've already mentioned as valuable tools to manage stress and improve sleep.

- **Light therapy (photobiomodulation or PBM).** Light in the red and near-infrared spectrum has been used for years to treat injuries and reduce inflammation in joints, on the skin, and in the body. In the last several years, researchers have begun to explore the benefits of using these light technologies on the brain. Science suggests that PBM supports brain health in several ways. In the short term, it stimulates the mitochondria in brain cells to produce more energy, increases blood flow to brain cells (delivering more oxygen and nutrients), and stimulates the waste-removal process via the glymphatic system.[16] Longer-lasting effects include producing more antioxidants, reducing inflammation within the brain, and stimulating self-repair processes such as forming new neurons and synapses (the connections between neurons).[17] Red light therapy is also considered very low risk.[18] A 2023 review of thirty-eight studies found that light therapy made a significant positive impact on cognitive function in patients with dementia, and a significantly bigger impact than other non-pharmacological therapies.[19] Many gyms and wellness centers now offer red light therapy; you can also purchase a device for use at home. Research suggests that the optimal wavelengths are 660 nm and 810 nm, that the light should be pulsed rather than continuous, and that the light penetrates the brain best when directed at the lower portion of the back of the skull.[20] Check out NovaaLab and Hooga for reasonably priced at-home options.

- **Audio therapy.** Similar to how light can stimulate the brain, sounds can, too. Researchers at MIT have started small pilot studies in humans in which participants are exposed to light and sound at frequencies that match the neuronal frequencies that stimulate gamma brain waves, which are found to be impaired in people with dementia and play a role in memory formation. While these studies are still small and preliminary, their initial findings show that the participants' brains experienced an increase in gamma waves. Those with cognitive impairment experienced better connectivity between brain regions and more consistent sleep—all with no major side effects.[21] (Look for the TED Talk "Could We Treat Alzheimer's with Light and Sound?") A larger body of research has found that listening to music, playing music, and being exposed to sound therapy have a broad range of neurological benefits, including reducing anxiety and nervous system stimulation and stimulating the waste removal functions of the glymphatic system, which researchers theorize may aid in the removal of amyloid protein.[22]

- **Vaccines to reduce dementia risk.** Half of those with Alzheimer's disease have high levels of the bacterium *P. gingivalis*, which most of us have in small amounts in our mouths, but it can be activated by the iron from the blood released from the gums during a dental procedure (such as scaling and surgery), and then carried throughout the body in the bloodstream.[23] This bacterium contributes to gum disease and inflammation, and it is associated with both cardiovascular disease and Alzheimer's. The biotech company Lighthouse Pharmaceuticals is currently in a Phase 2b clinical trial to assess the safety and efficacy of drugs known as protease inhibitors that work to specifically reduce the population and toxicity of *P. gingivalis* to prevent the onset of Alzheimer's. (For more information, visit lighthousepharma .com.) Other types of vaccines are also in development—as of this writing, Andrea Pfeifer's company AC Immune is in Phase 2 clinical trials to gauge the effectiveness and safety of a vaccine to prevent the formation of new plaques. "Our mission is to have the vaccine against Alzheimer's by 2029," she told me, admitting that it's a tough goal but, she thinks, a realistic one.

Surprisingly, other existing vaccines appear to be helpful in reducing Alzheimer's risk as well—namely, flu, pneumonia (for people over sixty-five), and shingles vaccines. The flu and pneumonia can trigger dormant viruses, particularly herpes simplex type 1 (responsible for cold sores) and herpes zoster (the cause of shingles—a risk for anyone who had chicken pox as a child), which can then contribute to the development of Alzheimer's. The shingles vaccine, in particular, is associated with a 15 percent reduction in risk of developing both Alzheimer's and Parkinson's.[24] Because shingles can be such a painful condition—with a potential for rashes and nerve pain that can last for weeks—it seems a win-win to get the vaccine.

BRAIN HEALTH: WHERE TO BEGIN

If you do one thing: Exercise, preferably with friends, and/or do things that require real focus

What's good for the heart is good for the brain, and, as I've said before, exercise is a silver bullet to increase brainspan, healthspan, and lifespan. As we covered in Chapter 4, resistance training in particular boosts the production of BDNF and new neuron and neuronal connections, so while walking is great, aim for at least two sessions of strength training per week (at a moderate intensity for you and your fitness levels). And when you take that walk, hike, or bike ride with a friend, you also reap the benefits of more social connection (another ingredient in the holistic recipe, which we'll cover in the next chapter). To really maximize your workout time, periodically weave in tasks that require brain power—such as listening to a podcast to learn something new. This approach is called dual-task training, and multiple studies show that it can improve cognition in those with mild or moderate dementia and prevent dementia in those who don't yet display symptoms.[25] Stacking your activities in this way helps you reap a lot of benefits at once. And when you do it with a friend or loved one, you also benefit from social connection.

If you're a total beginner: Cut way down on sugar, alcohol, and ultra-processed foods

I've shared how much I enjoy a glass of wine at the end of the day—and sometimes two. Researching this book has made me rethink that. While I don't see myself giving it up completely, I have cut back to only having one glass once or twice a week. Plus, I've since learned that the liver slows down starting at around age forty, making it harder to metabolize the alcohol.[26] Similarly, because sugar can promote the glycation of brain cells, it's vital to cut back on how much sugar you eat. In fact, a French study found that people with an APOE4 gene who regularly had an afternoon snack high in refined (and thus low-fiber) carbs, such as a cookie, cereal bar, or sweetened coffee drink, had a significantly higher risk of developing Alzheimer's than people with an APOE4 gene who had either a lower-carb afternoon snack or no snack at all.[27]

If you're already doing well and want to take it to the next level: Prioritize learning new skills

Learning keeps those neurons strong and forges new connections—especially if your new skill is meditation. Not only does meditation reduce stress, but it has also been shown to boost the effectiveness of networks within the brain and performance on tests of verbal memory and produce small but still significant changes in executive function.[28] If you're already meditating, learn a new language, musical instrument, or athletic pursuit that also challenges you mentally (such as ballroom dancing or sailing). Your brain will thank you.

AGELESS AGING HACKS TO SAFEGUARD YOUR BRAINSPAN

Practice gratitude

Studies have linked practicing gratitude to better brain health. Expressing appreciation not only has been shown in studies to lead to greater happiness, more positive emotions, and significantly better mental health, but also to increase activity in the areas of the brain related to empathy and social bonding. Practicing gratitude—whether in writing, thought, or prayer—drives us to appreciate the positive aspects of our lives, fueling positive emotions and happiness. Even if you are a natural-born pessimist, you can alter your mindset (more on this in just a moment), building more mental and emotional resilience.

Breathe for stress relief

Remember, distress is bad for your brainspan. A quick hack that Lisa Genova shared is a simple breathing technique to use anytime you're hit with something super stressful. To do it, breathe in through your nose to the count of four, hold it for one second, then breathe out through your nose to the count of four. Why does this work? "If you are in a fight-or-flight response, your body is saying run for your life, and you are likely trying to gulp in air through your mouth to fuel that flight. This is a lovely nine-second thing you can do to bring your body back into a state of safety." If you can, close your eyes before you do it, as your brain quiets down a lot without the visual input.

Try meditation apps

Yes, your cell phone can be a huge distraction, undermining focus. It can also help you develop more mental resilience and concentration and reduce your bad stress thanks to the many meditation apps that are available. Calm, Endel, and Headspace are user-friendly. Other good options include Insight Timer, Ten Percent Happier, and Buddhify. All of these apps make meditating as easy as deciding to do it and pressing a button.

Drink warm water with lemon first thing in the morning

Lisa Mosconi's favorite brain hack that she shares in *The XX Brain* is starting the day with a glass of warm water. I've been doing it for years. The warmth will open up your blood vessels, helping deliver hydration more efficiently into your cells. I add a squeeze of lemon, a natural diuretic that helps flush out toxins and other waste products in your body and is a source of vitamin C.

Stay hydrated all day long

The brain is 80 percent water. Even mild dehydration can impair your thinking, trigger a headache,[29] and even shrink brain volume. Make sure you're getting half of your body weight in ounces of water throughout the day—herbal tea counts toward this goal, but seltzer, soda, coffee, caffeinated tea, juice, and energy drinks definitely don't. And if you're exercising, which you likely are doing after reading about all the benefits, make sure there are electrolytes in the water or add them in through a supplement.

Exercise in nature

As effective as exercise is at keeping your brain strong, when you do it outside in a natural setting, those benefits are boosted. A small study that had students take a fifteen-minute walk either outside or inside found that those who ventured out-of-doors displayed improved performance on a cognitively challenging task as well as brainwave activity that is associated with working memory and attention—two results that those who walked inside did not experience.[30] We are part of nature, after all, and when we are out in it, a wide body of research suggests that our nervous system calms down, as do our thoughts.

Take care of your teeth and gums

As I've mentioned, the bacterium responsible for gum disease, *P. gingivalis*, is also frequently found in the brains of Alzheimer's patients. In fact, in one study, gingipains, a type of toxic enzyme secreted by *P. gingivalis*, were found in 96 percent of the fifty-three brain tissue samples studied, with higher levels detected in those with Alzheimer's disease.[31]

What does this mean? According to Mark I. Ryder, professor of periodontology at UCSF, "the presence of *P. gingivalis* increased the production of amyloid beta, the part of the amyloid plaques directly linked to Alzheimer's. Our study confirmed via animal testing that *P. gingivalis* can travel from the mouth to the brain and that the related gingipains can destroy brain neurons." Yet another study, published in the *European Journal of Epidemiology*, found that "preventing and treating periodontitis could contribute to controlling the global epidemic of dementia."[32]

So, make sure you brush and floss well every day, twice a day. You may also want to use a tongue scraper, which removes the same plaque that builds up on your teeth. One important caveat is that you don't want to use antibacterial mouthwash, because it wipes out both unfriendly and friendly bacteria. And your body and microbiome need those friendly bacteria for a variety of functions. So, better to stick with mouthwashes that are not antibacterial. Or you can just rinse your mouth with water and ditch the mouthwash altogether.

Invest in research to end
Alzheimer's disease and cognitive decline

We want to end this disease, and you can help make that happen. Several nonprofits are working hard to help fund research and researchers to find a cure for Alzheimer's disease. Getting involved at a local or national level through your own time and/or money is a good investment for your future as well as the future of your children and grandchildren. A few of the organizations you can check out include the Alzheimer's Association, BrightFocus Foundation, WomenAgainstAlzheimer's, UsAgainstAlzheimer's, Cure Alzheimer's Fund, Alzheimer's Research UK, and the American Brain Foundation. You can also contact your government representatives and demand they support more funding for Alzheimer's research.

10

PURPOSE AND CONNECTION

Many people are surprised to learn how incredibly impactful meaningful relationships and a sense of purpose are for your healthspan, brainspan, and even your lifespan. When it comes to ageless aging, the potential upsides of nurturing our relationships with friends and family and of finding new ways to bring purpose to our daily lives are too potent to leave on the table.

Our research at Age Wave has been on the cutting edge of exploring the impact that purpose and social capital have on our well-being as we live longer lives. In one of our 2023 studies with more than nine thousand adults, including more than seven hundred women fifty and over, we learned that as we live longer, the greatest source of purpose for most women is spending quality time with loved ones. These two elements—purpose and social capital—are closely linked.

Of course, besides spending time with family, there are lots of other ways to add meaning to your life, including living a spiritual or faith-filled life, which for many ranks high. Marc Freedman, a renowned social entrepreneur, thought leader, author, and founder and co-CEO of CoGenerate, told me about purpose with a little p and Purpose with a big P. Purpose with a little p can sometimes be as simple as enjoying walking your dog, babysitting your grandchild, or sharing a meal with friends. On the other hand, Purpose with a big P can be something as

244 ◆ AGELESS AGING

momentous as starting your own business, volunteering for a cause that makes your heart sing, or getting involved in an issue that can have a positive impact on the world at large.

In this chapter, I'll share the *why* of social connections and purpose as well as some strategies and tools for strengthening your sense of purpose and building your social community, which sometimes involve the exact same actions. But first, let's understand the importance of connection by looking at the growing epidemic of isolation and loneliness in our society, especially among older adults.

THE LONELINESS AND ISOLATION HEALTH CRISIS

Scientific data confirms the fact that loneliness has the same health risk as smoking fifteen cigarettes daily.[1] Research has linked loneliness to elevated inflammation and increased blood pressure, and even identified it as a contributor to heart disease, depression, and early death.[2] According to Dr. Dean Ornish, clinical professor of medicine at the University of California, San Francisco, and president and founder of the Preventive Medicine Research Institute, "thousands of studies show that people who are lonely and depressed are three to ten times more likely to get sick and die prematurely from pretty much all causes, when compared to those who have a sense of love, and connection, and community." He added, "It's partly through mechanisms we doctors don't fully understand."

While these data points have been known by researchers and social scientists for some time, it was the pandemic that brought this crisis to the forefront. With its extended lockdowns and the ushering in of an era of remote work and school and the very elderly being isolated in nursing homes, loneliness and isolation became more evident and more prominent. The silver lining—if there is one—is the wake-up call about the importance of social connection that caught our cultural attention.

In 2023, U.S. surgeon general Dr. Vivek Murthy labeled loneliness an epidemic, declaring: "Our relationships are a source of healing and well-being hiding in plain sight. Given the significant health consequences of loneliness and isolation, we must prioritize building social connections the same way we have prioritized other critical public health issues such as tobacco, obesity, and substance use disorders."

Loneliness is harmful at any age, and during the pandemic, young people were particularly vulnerable. But its presence and its perils can become more prominent as we live long lives. Historically, it wasn't always like that, as Dana Griffin, co-founder and CEO of Eldera.ai, the global platform for wisdom sharing and intergenerational connection, told me: "We evolved as a society with the old taking care of the young while the middle generation worked. We disrupted that connection with the invention of the nuclear family in the twentieth century." Dana further explained, "Now one in three older adults are lonely, and that goes up to 50 percent in people eighty and older. That has huge health ramifications."

The health boons from eliminating loneliness and isolation are significant. The importance of community on health and longevity has been confirmed in multiple seminal studies, including the Harvard Study of Adult Development and Dan Buettner's well-known Blue Zones research in areas of the world with the highest percentage of centenarians. In Blue Zones, generations tend to live closer to one another, belong to faith-based communities, have strong individual senses of purpose, and take part in communal meals with a glass of wine to enjoy each other's company.[3] In one of the Blue Zones, in Okinawa, people intentionally form "moais," which are small groups of about five friends who have committed to lifelong friendship and who meet on a daily or weekly basis. Often formed in early childhood, some moais have lasted over ninety years.

Harvard University's Study of Adult Development is the longest study of human happiness to date and reinforces the learnings from the Blue Zones research. In this eighty-years-and-counting ongoing investigation, they find that having supportive, positive relationships is the primary key to happiness, especially as we live longer. Study director Robert Waldinger, a psychology professor at Harvard Medical School, said in his TED Talk: "When we gathered together everything we knew about our study participants at age fifty, it wasn't their cholesterol levels that predicted how they were going to grow old. It was how satisfied they were in their relationships—the people who were the most satisfied in their relationships at age fifty were the healthiest at age eighty."[4]

WELLNESS STARTS WITH "WE"—ESPECIALLY FOR WOMEN

Chip Conley, founder of the Modern Elder Academy, told me, "We tend to get very fixated on individual wellness, but interestingly, the word *illness* starts with an *I*, and *wellness* starts with a 'we.'" There's actually a medical term for the social aspect of health; it's called social fitness. Conley shared another helpful way of thinking about it: "Community is a social safety net. We have property liability insurance for our home, but where's the emotional insurance for our personal rainy days?"

As we live longer, the need for stimulating social interactions and nourishing relationships becomes even stronger, particularly for women, because we are more likely to live alone as we age. Once we reach sixty-five, women in the United States are twice as likely as men to live alone either because they've been widowed (due to superior longevity) or because they have chosen to live solo.[5] Either way, this can make women more vulnerable than men to the negative effects of isolation and loneliness.

That said, you don't have to be a social butterfly with hundreds of people in your circle. You also don't have to have a big group of best friends. While quantity matters somewhat, the depth of our relationships matters even more.

"It's nice to have a good mix of both strong and weak ties," Dr. Kelli Harding, psychiatrist, assistant professor of psychiatry at Columbia University Medical Center, and author of *The Rabbit Effect*, explained. That means the interactions you have when you go to the coffee shop or the grocery store or say hi to your neighbor who's down the street are little bits of daily connection that add up to something meaningful. "I recommend to all of my patients that they be really intentional about developing those relationships across the board."

Helen Dennis, one of the pioneers in the field of aging, is a retirement coach, the syndicated columnist of "Successful Aging," and is herself in her eighties. She has been widowed for more than twenty years. When she speaks about relationships, she does so as both an expert and a woman who actively works to build her own social network. She offers this advice: "When it comes to relationships, I think it's important at this later life stage that we learn to take the initiative. It takes practice, because not everyone is a natural initiator."

Ultimately, you want to try to have a diverse portfolio of relationships. "Many of the studies that have been done around immune system functioning have shown that people who have a broader range of friendships actually fare better," Dr. Harding said. However, while virtual connections can be helpful, they can't be everything. "It's important to share physical space with people," Dr. Harding said, so that you can read their body language and do what psychologists call co-regulating—matching our moods and emotions to the people around us, something we've done since infancy without perhaps being conscious of it.

Do a social inventory. Ask yourself, "Do I regularly talk to people during the day? Have I made time to connect with a loved one today?" If the answer is no to either of these questions, it's time to get out there, or, if you are homebound, invite folks in. It's worth mentioning that if the people you are relating to *don't* make you feel accepted, supported, or safe—or their presence makes you feel stressed, judged, or unimportant—they are toxic. While every relationship will have its ups and downs, if a relationship feels toxic, consider how to protect yourself by talking it through, minimizing your contact with that person, or ending the relationship altogether.

KINDNESS FOSTERS SOCIAL FITNESS

Kindness is so powerful a health intervention that Dr. Harding said, "I wish I could prescribe kindness to all of my patients because it's one of those things where there's very little downside and a huge potential gain."

Giving kindness reduces cortisol,[6] blood pressure,[7] and premature causes of death.[8] And it doesn't have to be a grand gesture or a lifetime of selfless service. Even small acts of kindness, or what Dr. Harding called micro-kindnesses, can have an impact. These are things like making eye contact, smiling, reaching out to someone, offering a helping hand when you notice something, or stepping in when you see that somebody's in a hard situation.[9]

Not only do these simple acts benefit you, but they can also have a ripple effect. "Studies show that when you do a small act of kindness, it inspires the person who's on the receiving end to do an act of kindness in return, and it also inspires whoever is watching the act of kindness to pay it forward," Dr. Harding shared. Best of all, giving kindness costs nothing and doesn't take much time at all. I've included more on micro-kindnesses in the hacks section of this chapter so that you can start incorporating it—and reaping the benefits—right away.

WAKE-UP CALL FOR SOLO AGERS

Since relationships and social fitness are so vitally important, if we're not married/partnered or don't have close family ties, what do we do? Dr. Sara Zeff Geber, PhD, author of *Essential Retirement Planning for Solo Agers*, is a certified retirement coach and a leading expert on solo aging. She has a broad definition of solo aging: anyone who is getting older who doesn't have a partner or family support, including those who never had children, or who are estranged from their children or other family members. It's a surprisingly large number of people—almost 20 percent of boomer women never had children, and that percentage will surely rise in younger generations as the number of women opting out of motherhood grows.

Dr. Zeff Geber became interested in solo aging in her sixties, when one of her good friends spent the better part of a year flying across the country helping her mom move out of her home and into an assisted living facility. "I don't have kids, and my friend also doesn't have kids. I looked at her and said, 'Who's going to do that for us?' Neither of us had a clue." It was a wake-up call for Dr. Zeff Geber to help herself—and others in her position—strengthen connections and social fitness.

While all of us can be vulnerable to isolation and loneliness, solo agers need to more proactively take steps to ward off the negative health impacts of isolation, and for practical reasons. Who will pick you up after your colonoscopy appointment or other medical procedure and care for you when you aren't able to care for yourself? Whose name will you write down on your "in case of emergency" forms to help make decisions when you aren't able to do so on your own? Dr. Zeff Geber told me her biggest piece of advice for solo agers is, "Live in community. We solo agers need to be even more intentional about building community. What that looks like depends on your particular pocketbook, but there are many more options than you might think." Just think back to that classic television show *Golden Girls* to see that finding a roommate or two, or creating some kind of communal living or meal-sharing experience, can add a strong sense of community to your life.

STEPPING UP YOUR SOCIAL FITNESS GAME

While it's true that solo agers have more direct challenges to consider than those who are partnered or have children, chances are your children may live far away, like mine do. My son, Zak, and his wife, FeyFey, live in Shanghai, and my daughter, Casey, lives in Los Angeles. Yes, we're all close, make a huge effort to see each other often, and I'm lucky to get to speak to them almost daily via Zoom or phone, but I recognize the importance of having a social circle outside of my relationship with them and with my husband, Ken.

Dr. Zeff Geber suggests joining a religious community, such as a church, synagogue, mosque, or ashram, even if you aren't religious. A good friend of mine, Rick, and his wife, Linda, recently moved from Los Angeles, where they had a large group of lifelong friends, to San Diego to be closer to their children and grandchildren. The upside was getting to spend more time with the grandchildren; the downside was having to start over to build community. Linda told me, "It was great to be with my grandchildren so much, but I really missed my friends. I'm not a very religious person, but I joined a church that held get-togethers for new members. I'm not really a joiner, but I needed a way to meet people and create bonds in the community. So we joined, and we were lucky enough to meet a lot of great people. As corny as it might sound, Rick and I started 'friend dating' and we developed a few really meaningful couple friendships. It really helped provide a feeling of community, and just made us happier."

There are all kinds of adult-oriented networking groups, book clubs, and classes popping up everywhere that can lead to new friendships. If you don't find one that feels right, start your own. That's what Helen Dennis did. It started with a conversation with her friend Bernice Bratter, who had just retired. Bernice asked Helen, "Is there anything available for career women moving into retirement? Where is the research? Where are the programs?" Helen said, "Bernice, we are *not* on the radar."

These two women changed that reality. It started with each of them inviting a handful of women to join them for dinner to discuss the transition into retirement and how to make it purposeful. What evolved from that was a monthly meeting at Bernice's home. They would pick a topic that was relevant for career women who felt passionate about their work and were moving into what they labeled "this empty wasteland called retirement." It was all about *Who am I without my business card?* Or *What does productivity mean in this life stage?* This led to Project Renewment (renewment.org), which spread by word of mouth throughout the country with both virtual and in-person events. Helen told me, "The impact that we had was not anticipated. We inadvertently created small, enduring communities of women that have been meeting anywhere from two to twenty-three years." Eventually, Bernice turned their learnings into a book that was a *Los Angeles Times* bestseller. This is a perfect example of combining purpose and social connections.

In Age Wave's 2023 study "Resilient Choices," done in partnership with the Harris Poll and Edward Jones, we learned that adopting a dog had a tremendous impact on boosting one's sense of purpose. It's also a popular and successful way to meet others and build relationships. That may sound like a cliché, but anytime you're walking a dog, you're going to meet people—people who want to pet your dog, or other dog owners. One of my friends, Lyndsey, who has never been married, moved from Marin County to Sonoma County when she stopped working full-time because the cost of living was so much more reasonable. As a solo ager, she was intent on building community. She told me, "When I was house-hunting, I looked around to see which neighborhoods seemed to have people walking their dogs. When I did move, my dog was the key to my building a close-knit friendship network. I got to know all the other people who were walking their dog in the neighborhood every day at five o'clock. We started planning potluck dinners together, then we went to the movies or wine tasting, and eventually it became a thriving social network. When I had knee surgery, my neighbors were the ones who helped me out in every possible way. My dog, who is a rescue, has really rescued me."

LOVE AND ROMANCE

Not surprisingly, an important source of connection is romantic relationships, whether you're already partnered, dating, or dreaming about finding love and romance. The longer we live, the more diverse our long-term relationships are. One potential challenge in romantic relationships among older adults is work status—if one partner is retired, or wants to retire, while the other wants or needs to keep working, it can be a big hurdle to that relationship.

As I mentioned earlier, Helen Dennis lost her husband more than twenty years ago. Ten years later, she reconnected with a man she had dated in college. The two realized they still cared about each other and had a lot in common, so they began dating. "For seven years, we had a long-distance relationship—he'd come here to California from the East Coast for a couple weeks, and then I'd go visit him. We traveled together. It was perfect." Ultimately, it was not perfect for him. The gist of the problem was that he was fully retired, while Helen was still enjoying work. "He wanted a full-time woman," she observed. In the end, even though they were the same age, "we were at different life stages." That doesn't mean it was easy to break up. "It was a big loss for me," she said. Helen tried dating again, but "I was so underwhelmed." She's taken herself off the market. "I love men, no question, but I'm content on my own." Helen actually does have a new man in her life—her eighteen-year-old grandson, who's temporarily living with her. "It's a joy to see the world through his eyes and we have so much fun together."

Navigating work-life balance with a romantic partner isn't something that just goes away because you're at an age where you're eligible for Social Security. When I interviewed Dr. Carol Kuhle of Mayo Clinic, she shared that she had just gotten married. I asked her, "What's it like to start a new relationship as an independent professional woman in her sixties?" She said that although they were very compatible, with common interests—they met at the gym, and it turned out they both lived in the same condo complex—they have had to put a lot of thought and effort into creating the right balance of time spent together versus time spent focused on work. "I told him, you're getting a professional woman with a demanding job."

Blending families can be complicated even when your children are fully grown, and Dr. Kuhle advises against rushing into making a relationship permanent. "Try to just get to know each other over time, be open, and seek to create intimacy—because sexual health is very important at any age," Kuhle said.

Kuhle is not alone. Many women find love, romance, and companionship in their fifties, sixties, and beyond. And not all of them move slowly. My dad passed away suddenly at age sixty, leaving my mom, who had been with my dad since they were in high school, devastated, grieving, and alone. About two years later, at age sixty herself, my mom, who had never even dated anyone other than my dad, began dating.

About six months after that, I got a call from my mom, who told me she was in love. Not surprisingly, I was in shock, and said to my mom, "You just started dating. This could just be a rebound from

Dad's death." I then asked her when she'd met the guy, to which she responded, "Two days ago. And I'd really like you to come meet him. By the way, he just moved in with me. Oh, and his name is Ray."

A two-day romance culminating in a move-in? My mom was a very buttoned-up woman, and I immediately thought she'd gone a little crazy. And who was this Ray guy? After I gathered my wits, I reached out to my brother Richard, a lawyer, who was already setting in motion a criminal record search on Ray. We were all alarmed, believing it was possible that she was being bamboozled.

But she wasn't. My mom and Ray had fallen in love. And Ray turned out to be a loving, caring man whose first wife had passed away decades earlier from cancer. The following year, we celebrated their love with a glorious wedding at our home, attended by their friends, their adult children and children-in-law (thirteen), their grandchildren (lots), and even two great-grandchildren.

Since my mom was in her sixties and Ray was in his early seventies, they didn't get married to have kids. They did not get married to pursue their careers. They got married to enjoy each other. And they did—with both of them feeling that the second time around they had found the true love of their lives.

Of course, if you've been married for a long time, like I have been, you have to work to maintain and grow your relationship continually. This requires commitment, vision, and a little imagination. One strategy that Ken and I have adopted to keep our bond of love strong is to renew our wedding vows every single year. Not only do we renew our vows, but we also review our relationship and try to find ways to make it even better and more resilient.

We got married (the first time) in a small, intimate ceremony followed by a celebration with close family and friends in our home in Berkeley, officiated by the two singing rabbis of Marin County. We intentionally chose to have our marriage on Thanksgiving Day. We agreed that getting married on a day of thanks made enormous sense because we both felt such gratitude to have found each other and to have the opportunity to build a life and a family together. During the celebration, Ken turned to me and said, "This is so much fun, we should do it every year."

I loved the idea. To add a little spice, we decided that we'd go to a different location and get married by a different individual or religious entity each year. At this writing, we've been married more than forty times—by a Presbyterian minister on the cliffs of Kona, a judge accompanied by a mariachi band in Cabo San Lucas, a minister at the Chapel of Love in Las Vegas, the skiing judge of Vail, a Buddhist monk in our home, and even by our kids . . . just to name a few. It's a way for us to punctuate the moment and our deep love and respect for each other. We talk about what went on for us that year—the highs, the lows, and what we want to do differently this upcoming year. It's been a lot of fun, but also an important touchstone to keep us growing, learning, and building resilience in our relationship. We also get to clear the air, realign, and reprioritize our love for each other. One year we delayed our renewal ceremony for a few months—it was a particularly hectic and stressful year—and it had a negative effect on our relationship. We've never put it off again.

ANOTHER CONNECTION
TO NURTURE—YOUR PURPOSE

Another key component of healthspan and lifespan is having a sense of purpose. By now, you've probably connected the dots and noticed the direct link between social connections and purpose. In fact, one of the seminal findings in a recent Age Wave study was that 92 percent of retirees—women and men—agree that purpose is key to a successful retirement and that family is the number-one way many of us feel a sense of purpose.[10]

While a sense of purpose has always been recognized as important, it is an increasingly important area of exploration in terms of longer healthspan and lifespan. In 1946, Viktor Frankl wrote the classic book *Man's Search for Meaning*, on concentration camp survivors. A trained psychiatrist who was imprisoned in Nazi Germany, he wrote about how it wasn't necessarily the youngest, the healthiest, or the strongest individuals who survived. It was those who could find meaning and purpose in their lives even in that horrific experience. The vital takeaway is that we have the power to choose our mindset even in the worst of circumstances.

The most recent scientific research proves Viktor Frankl was right: lack of a sense of purpose can lead to shorter healthspans and lifespans.[11] The flip side of that coin, according to Alan Rozanski, a professor at the Icahn School of Medicine at Mount Sinai, is that "the need for meaning and purpose is the deepest driver of well-being there is." In a 2021 Age Wave study on purpose, 87 percent of women surveyed said that "being useful made them feel more youthful."[12] Clearly, purpose is a key ingredient in our holistic recipe for ageless aging.

Health Benefits of Having a Strong Sense of Purpose

Having a strong sense of purpose reduces risk of:[13]

- Alzheimer's
- Cardiovascular problems
- Depression
- Stroke
- Disability

Those with a higher sense of purpose have:

- Better overall health
- Greater cognitive functioning
- Higher life satisfaction
- Increased mobility/functioning
- Longer lifespans

Having a sense of purpose has been linked to consciously extending an individual's lifespan. "When I talk to other doctors, everyone has a story about a patient with a grim prognosis who really wanted to make it to a child's wedding or the birth of a child or a birthday, and did it despite all odds," Dr. Harding told me. "That's incredible agency." My mother-in-law, Pearl, really wanted to make it to her ninety-third birthday. We all traveled to Florida to celebrate with her, and she had been looking forward to it for months. But her entire system was breaking down: she was really suffering from Alzheimer's, COPD, and heart disease, and could barely get out of bed. However, she made it to her birthday celebration, dressing for the occasion with a big smile, and passed away just a few days later.

These may seem like extreme examples, but the fact is that purpose is an essential success factor in living a long life. Equally importantly, purpose can help us maintain our vitality, energy, and wellness longer. Dr. Linda Fried, head of Columbia University's Mailman School of Public Health, told me, "I have seen patient after patient, older adults, who came to me because they felt sick. What I found was that the reason they felt sick was they had no reason to get up in the morning." As a result, one of the most common prescriptions Fried writes for her retired patients is "Find your purpose."

Common Sources of Purpose

Individual forms of purpose

Family

Faith

Pets

Work, volunteering, or "menterning"

Grief (channeling loss into a meaningful project)

> Hobbies (such as growing a garden, researching your ancestry, or writing a book)
>
> Social and community groups (such as book clubs, fitness groups, or networking groups)
>
> **Collective forms of purpose**
>
> Legacy
>
> Passing your wisdom along
>
> Making the world a better place in some small way

WORK CAN HELP DEFINE YOUR PURPOSE

As we live longer, work is something many of us may choose to keep doing, in part to create a sense of purpose. For instance, I'm seventy-three years old, and I love my work. If I were to stop, it would create a huge void. However, my husband, Ken, and I are now trying to create a new work-life balance by taking off more time to play.

One of the silver linings of the pandemic was that new ways to work became more accepted, such as working from home or a hybrid approach that involved working a couple of days at home and a couple of days in the office. The four-day workweek, working ten hours a day, also gained some traction, with studies showing that it boosted employee morale and productivity. These types of innovations make it easier to find balance between work and other life pursuits.

You may enjoy your career and either stay in the same firm at which you already worked, try a different job, or create your own business. It may mean working full-time, part-time, or flex-time. Through the research conducted at Age Wave, 59 percent of people forty-five and older surveyed said the ideal plan for the next stage of life was to work in some form, be it full-time, part-time, or flex-time.

In yet another Age Wave study, we probed deeper into the benefits of working beyond the traditional retirement age of sixty-five. We asked pre-retirees what they expected to miss most about work once they stopped. The top thing they mentioned was reliable income, which makes a lot of sense. But when we asked retirees what they actually missed most about work, it wasn't the money. It was the social connections. Again, social connection and purpose are tightly linked for most of us.

GIVING BACK GIVES BACK

Another valuable tool for creating a sense of purpose in life is giving back in its many shapes and forms. "Many older adults have more than a desire—they have a *need* to feel that they've left their corner of the world better than they found it," Fried explained to me. Volunteering your time, even if it's just a few hours a week, to a cause that really matters to you is a win for you and a win for the world at large. What we've learned in our Age Wave research is that once women are retired, they are more likely to volunteer *if* they had started the habit of volunteering before they retired. We also learned that those who do volunteer report feeling significantly healthier and happier with a greater sense of purpose.

Lynne Twist, seventy-eight years old at this writing, an author, activist, and one of the founders of the Hunger Project, the Pachamama Alliance, and the Soul of Money Institute, is a woman who has made this idea of leaving the world a better place her life's mission. In 1977, Lynne was one of the founders of the Hunger Project, whose mission was to end world hunger in twenty-five years. She traveled throughout the world, setting up grassroots organizations to help poorer communities become self-sufficient in terms of growing and making available their own food. It has been a model for many other nonprofits to help end world hunger. Lynne told me she doesn't believe in charity; rather, she believes in empowerment. She went on to be the founder of the Pachamama Alliance, whose mission is "to empower indigenous people of the Amazon rainforest to preserve their lands and culture."

Lynne explained to me, "It's such an epic time to be alive. There's so much to do. So much to transform and accomplish. Giving back, in the twenty-first century, is about solidarity. It's about realizing everybody has gifts, everybody has something to offer, everybody has a unique role to play." Lynne added, "If I know that I'm making a difference with my life, with my day, with my time, then I'm happy. I like to see what's mine to do."

We women are an invaluable natural resource that needs to be wisely put to work to help create a better world for our children and grandchildren. No longer can we as a society afford to lose the time and wisdom of hundreds of millions of women as we live longer. We need to take a stand and be counted on to make the world a better place—and also gain more health and vitality in the process.

CUTTING-EDGE APPROACHES
TO CONNECTION AND PURPOSE

- **Modern Elder Academy (MEA).** Chip Conley has created an innovative program for women and men fifty and older to rediscover their sense of purpose, providing the structure, support, and a gorgeous environment to make it possible for you to ponder the big questions about where you are and where you want to go. Kerry Hannon, a friend, author, and personal finance editor for Yahoo, recently attended as a guest teacher and told me that it was life-changing. One of the biggest benefits was that she made lasting friendships with other participants, people who value the same things she does, including finding renewed purpose. MEA holds in-person classes and retreats on its Baja, Mexico, campus, and they are building another campus near Santa Fe, New Mexico, as I write this; they also have virtual learning options at their website, modernelderacademy.com. Conley tells me that 62 percent of their students are women, which suggests that we women are hungry for adding more meaning to our lives.

- **Eldera.** Eldera (Eldera.ai) is all about intergenerational connection and the transmission of wisdom and life lessons from elders to children and back again. Co-founder Dana Griffin explains, "We're told to go out and search for our purpose, especially as we live longer, but the truth is we already have at least one essential purpose: to transmit our human wisdom—social [and] emotional skills, collaboration skills, the stories and traditions that got us this far—to the next generation." Eldera provides this outlet, matching vetted elders with kids for weekly virtual conversations and mentoring at scale. For example, my husband, Ken, referred a friend, Mary Ellen Klee, an acupuncturist from Los Angeles who is in her eighties, to Eldera. She had this to say about her experience:

> It occurred to me that I have never told you how much your turning me on to Eldera has enhanced my life. They matched me with a sixteen-year-old Haitian living in Miami who is just the most fabulous young woman. We talk weekly. She is always so excited to talk to me, and she has brightened my life and expanded my heart in more ways than I can say. She is a wonder with a "no limits" future. This is the best referral anybody has ever given me!

As Klee's testimony suggests, young people benefit from social-emotional learning and increased resilience, while older adults benefit from a sense of purpose and community. Everyone wins.

- **Center for Advanced Leadership at Harvard.** While this has been around for a while, it's a cutting-edge concept to create real transformation in the world. If you're interested in gaining the skills to unlock your potential to help solve some of the world's challenges, this one-year program might be perfect. You have to apply to the program, which utilizes many Harvard professors and departments to create an interdisciplinary curriculum emphasizing leadership development designed to help you create a social impact strategy for whatever issues you want to tackle. Plus you have full access to the Harvard community and the chance to create relationships with other like-minded people who are part of the program.

- **University-based retirement communities.** If you're a lifelong learner and lover of campus life, you can meet your need for community, keep your brain sharp, and foster intergenerational friendships by moving into a retirement community located on a college campus. As I write this, there are approximately a hundred university-based retirement communities in thirty states, where residents can easily partake in classes, lectures, sports events, and even research. Many also provide access to assisted living, skilled nursing, and memory care should the need arise. Universities win by gaining a new revenue stream, which is an important way to counteract declining enrollment due to this generation of college kids being smaller than in previous years. Stanford, Duke, Notre Dame, and the University of Alabama are just a few of the schools that host such communities. To investigate this option, do an internet search for "university-based retirement communities."

PURPOSE AND CONNECTION: WHERE TO BEGIN

If you do one thing: Try volunteering, even if it's just for an hour a week

There are so many ways you can make the world a better place and improve your own life at the same time. Whether it's at the local dog rescue, tutoring program, food bank, or wherever your personal interests take you, they need your help. Call, sign up, and just do it. The bonus is, along the way, you're sure to forge relationships with others who have similar interests.

If you're a beginner: Break up with toxic friends

If someone in your life is continuously making you feel bad about yourself, gaslighting you, or just making you unhappy, try communicating your concerns to them. If that doesn't bring positive change, spend less time with that person or put that relationship on pause. You may be surprised how much better you feel.

If you're ready to take it to the next level: Find a class at your local community college that piques your interest, and make friends with one or more of your classmates

Remember when you were growing up, you made friends at school? It was the same thing when you were in college, right? Now is the time to revisit this method of making friends. Local community colleges are a great resource for classes for adults of all ages. If you love art or music, or if you want to learn to play pickleball, chances are your local community college has a class that meets your needs. And it will be filled with people who have a similar interest. It's an opportunity to stimulate your brain, learn something new, find purpose, and expand your social network. Now that's a real win.

AGELESS AGING HACKS TO FOSTER PURPOSE AND CONNECTION

Keep working

"The evidence is clear that spending thirty years—the final third of your life—in nonworking retirement isn't good for the individual or for society," Dr. Fried told me. For the individual, the lack of stimulation and isolation are vitality killers. According to Dr. Fried, "People who retire and do nothing get sick and have greater healthcare needs. In addition, they aren't contributing to our collective wisdom." A study at the University of Michigan found a direct link between continued work and longevity when it concluded that people who work past the age of sixty-five add years to their life.[14] It can be a great tool for reinvention to find a new career path, turn a hobby into a side hustle, or start a business working part-time, flex-time, or as much as you'd like. Work has been proven to help keep you vital, socially connected, and worrying less about money. There is one caveat: don't continue working in ways that can burn out your physical or mental health.

Be a joiner

It's so easy for your world—and your worldview—to slowly get smaller as you live longer. But, as Helen Dennis told me, "we have to have some sense of self-responsibility—no one is stopping us from putting ourselves out there except us." Join a book club or a class to learn something new, or try one of these organizations: Generations Over Dinner (generationsoverdinner.com), which, as I mentioned earlier in the book, organizes meals where people of all ages get together and discuss the deeper meaning of life; Project Renewment (referenced earlier); and Third Act, which mobilizes older adults to get involved in climate change advocacy (thirdact.org). There are also language schools, art centers, community theater groups, and even community colleges where you can find your people as you learn.

Do an act of micro-kindness

"Doing something kind is a very fast way to turn around a lousy mood or a lousy day," Dr. Harding shared with me when I asked if she had any hacks for boosting well-being. Her favorite quick kindness is to pick up three pieces of trash around her New York City neighborhood. "If I'm in a grumpy mood, it works like magic." By doing this, she has inspired her neighbors to do the same, and they have created neighborhood clean-up days that have led to closer friendships as well as cleaner streets.

Be bold and take the initiative

Reach out to the friend you haven't spoken to in months—or years—or strike up a conversation with someone new. Helen Dennis shared a story with me about how she was at a movie by herself and realized she was sitting next to a woman from her synagogue. Although the two women didn't know each other, this woman's husband had been Helen's internist, and he had died a few months earlier. Helen, a widow herself, knew how isolating this could be, and so she said, "You don't know me, but your husband was my doctor. Do you enjoy going to the theater?" The woman said yes, and Helen asked if she would like to be theater buddies. It was the start of what blossomed into a lovely friendship, all because Helen was bold.

Get a manicure, massage, or other treatments that involve human touch

Really. Adding kind, supportive touch into your life, especially if you're a solo ager, is important. "Things like a manicure or a massage may seem like luxuries, but they're a form of physical connection, and the data says that touch is really critical to our well-being," Harding told me.

Travel with your grandchildren

Traveling with grandchildren, also known as gramping, is a win-win-win: you get special time with your grandchildren, you free up your children to focus on their lives and work or just get some time together without the kids, and, of course, you get to deepen your bond with your grandchildren. There are all kinds of programs at national parks, for instance, that cater specifically to gramping. There are also gramping cruises and tours. Check out Road Scholar at roadscholar.org.

Renew your wedding vows

If you're in a long-term relationship with a partner/spouse, renew your wedding vows. You can combine it with a vacation or just do it at a local park. The point is to acknowledge your relationship as being important enough to revisit your vows and maybe even think about how you might improve that relationship. You don't want a long-term relationship to grow stale on autopilot.

11

---◆---

THE WEALTH-HEALTH CONNECTION

What really makes your ageless aging recipe a complete meal is financial well-being. When you have your financial house in order, it impacts your health in so many positive ways, lowering your stress and anxiety and improving your peace of mind. It also gives you the physical and emotional bandwidth to pursue your interests, whether it's learning a new language, volunteering your time, exploring a new career, spending more time with family and friends, pursuing travel, or doing just about anything that makes your heart sing.

No matter how old you are or how you've related to money in the past, it's never too late to add this ingredient to your holistic recipe for ageless aging. Frankly, if you're going to live well into your eighties or nineties, or even to a hundred, you're going to need financial knowhow, confidence, and a plan for how to fund all those extra years of life. The financial aspect of longevity is uncharted territory, as even the financial services industry often assumes you'll retire at sixty-five and live to only eighty. But you can get there with a sense of discovery, a willingness to increase your money knowledge, and confidence.

It's time for each of us to step up to the plate and take financial responsibility for our lives today as well as plan for our future selves. When I spoke to Kerry Hannon, financial expert and prolific author, she put it bluntly: "You've got to take control of your money future—no one's going to do it for you." If that thought makes you shake in your shoes, take a deep breath and dive in. Implementing the tips in this chapter can help increase your confidence in your ability to manage money, and that confidence is a key part of success.

First, let's take a look at what we really mean when we use the word *wealth*.

WEALTH IS ACTUALLY ABOUT WELL-BEING

Wealth is a loaded word that conjures up images of excess and privilege, but "the etymology of the word *wealth* has nothing to do with money," Lynne Twist, author of *The Soul of Money*, explained to me. Rather, it is derived from Old English and means "well-being," which, Twist told me, means "having access to the 'well of being' that never runs out." In other words, wealth is having an abundance of wellness.

You don't need to be rich to be wealthy, though money certainly can help. The question is, how can you take care of your money so that it takes care of you on your hundred-year life path? After all, money isn't an end in itself, but it is an essential ingredient in the recipe for ageless aging that impacts all the other ingredients.

CHARTING THE FINANCIAL CONSEQUENCES
OF WOMEN'S LIFE JOURNEY

Knowledge is power, so let's take a look at how each step along women's life journey impacts our financial realities. Before you get discouraged, understand that there are solutions to each of these challenges. We'll get to them. But if we don't clearly recognize we face the challenges to begin with, we'll be caught in a far more difficult circumstance than if we acknowledge them and plan accordingly.

In the simplest terms possible: On average, women live about six years longer than men and retire about two years earlier than men. As a result, we spend more years in retirement than men. Women now graduate from college and complete grad school in higher numbers than men, which is a historic positive flip-flop that provides us with better career opportunities. Yet it comes at a cost in the form of more student debt, as women are currently responsible for 58 percent of all student debt.[1] We also are more likely than men to take time out of the workforce to take care of children, grandchildren, parents, and in-laws as they, too, live longer. Since women in mixed-gender relationships often marry men a little older than they are, we are also likely to be caring for a partner/spouse in our later years. In fact, the average woman spends 44 percent of her adult life out of the workforce, often in a caregiving role, compared to 28 percent for a man.[2]

This time spent caring for people we love can make for a varied, rich, and rewarding life, but it also comes with financial consequences. On average, women only have 70 percent as much money in our retirement accounts as men do.[3] Even more concerning, the Census Bureau reports that a full half of women ages fifty-five to sixty-six have no retirement savings at all.[4] While Social Security is an essential piece of your financial puzzle once you hit retirement age, you definitely don't want to be financially dependent on it alone, as inflation, state taxes, and an uncertain political future may chip away at it.

These realities can be unsettling, to say the least. Yet understanding how the circumstances of each life stage impact your financial security makes it possible to plan for these eventualities in advance. And when you can plan, obstacles become more manageable, surmountable, and—even better—preventable.

THINKING LIKE A BREADWINNER

There's no doubt that women have come a long way. In 1982, women earned only 65 cents on the dollar compared to men. By 2002, our earnings were up to 80 cents. That pay gap has continued to narrow, albeit not by much. According to the Pew Research Center, in 2022 U.S. women earned an average of 82 cents to a man's dollar.[5] Analysis by the Center for American Progress determined that, at the rate we're going, the pay gap won't fully close until 2056.[6]

These numbers don't fully land until you calculate the amount of money those missing pennies add up to over the course of a lifetime. Hold on to your jaw, because over a forty-year career, that average pay gap adds up to a staggering $590,000.[7] As high as this number is, it still doesn't account for the years that women spend out of the workforce caregiving.

In today's world of easy credit and online banking, it's easy to forget that women were shut out of much financial life until recently. "Let's face it, money is power, and women historically haven't had access to money," Ric Edelman, author, podcaster, and founder of Edelman Financial Services, told me. In the not-so-distant past, women couldn't open a bank account, let alone an investment account. Early in my lifetime, women couldn't have a credit card without their husband or father cosigning. We've made enormous strides we should be proud of. But there's still more work to be done.

First, women need to invest more in themselves and their careers. Graduating from college and completing grad school in such high numbers is a tremendous leap forward. We need to take this further and make sure we're negotiating the best possible salary and benefits package again and again. Find out what others in the field and the company you're planning on working in are making, and bust the pay gap. If you're already working, look your boss in the eye and ask for that promotion, that raise, and negotiate for perks such as stock options, royalties, and commissions. Men do this all the time, and we can follow their lead. Recognize that if we receive lower and fewer raises and take more time away from work to care for loved ones, it means we'll also receive less Social Security, 401(k) matching, and paid time off, which is not a good recipe for financial success.

Traditionally, most women have been socialized to think about earning money to pay their bills—not to build wealth and financial peace of mind. Jennifer Barrett, head of content for Fidelity Investments and author of *Think Like a Breadwinner*, says, "Women need to start looking at every paycheck that comes in as an opportunity to become less dependent on the next one." I think of it as funding your future self as well as your present self.

We also need to invest more in the financial markets. In Age Wave's study "Women and Money: Beyond the Bottom Line," the women surveyed told us that their biggest financial regret was not investing more money. According to a CNBC survey, 34 percent of white women, 48 percent of Hispanic women, and 59 percent of Black women have no financial investments at all.[8] None! The result is that white women own only 56 percent of the wealth that white men do. For Hispanic women, it's 10 percent. And Black women, only 5 percent.[9] We need to change this dynamic now.

On top of all this, research has found that women spend more on healthcare than men do, especially as they live longer—something I'll unpack shortly.

OWNING OUR COLLECTIVE FINANCIAL STRENGTHS

The outlook for women and their money is far from one of doom and gloom. We women possess multiple financial superpowers that provide a great foundation for us to build on. Remind yourself of these whenever your financial confidence needs bolstering.

- **We are on an upswing in terms of investing.** The percentage of women who invest beyond their retirement account is on the rise—67 percent in 2021, up from 44 percent in 2018.[10]
- **We are confident in most areas of financial decision-making except investing.** The Age Wave study "Women and Money: Beyond the Bottom Line" found that women are equally as confident as men when it comes to many financial tasks, such as paying bills (90 percent) and budgeting (84 percent). Yet only about half (52 percent) of women say they are confident in managing investments, compared to 68 percent of men—the largest gap (16 percent) between the sexes of any of the specific financial

tasks that we surveyed. Our basic comfort with making financial decisions is there; we only need to expand that existing comfort zone to include investing.

- **We gain better returns.** Women investors get higher returns, on average, than male investors, according to an analysis by Fidelity Investments as well as a University of California, Berkeley, study.[11] Although we may lack confidence around investing, we also don't suffer from overconfidence, which can color your view and make a so-so or even risky investment look like a good idea.

- **We are more patient.** Women tend to trade less frequently than men—up to 50 percent less, according to Vanguard.[12] That's good, because making a lot of trades is often counterproductive: getting in and out of more trades has been shown to reduce returns.[13]

- **We are less reactive.** When the market does crash, women tend not to react with extreme measures. A 2022 Nationwide survey found that after a market crash, only 8 percent of women sell off their retirement investments, compared to 15 percent of men.[14] Vanguard also found that women log into their investment accounts about 50 percent less often than men do, which means less temptation to buy or sell.

- **We wield a strong inner compass.** Women make more value-based financial decisions, considering what matters most to us, the people we care about, and the life we want to live. According to Age Wave studies, two-thirds of women want to invest in causes they care about and are primarily motivated to save and invest to take care of their families. Overall, we women take action to meet a goal like funding our children's education or providing care for a loved one rather than just reaching a particular number or showing off. We think of others, and we stay the course. That doesn't mean we don't care about financial performance: we do that, too.

I hope that with these elements laid out so clearly, it's getting into your head that we women have the necessary building blocks for improving our financial well-being. Now let's put them to work.

CHANGING THE NARRATIVE

While many of the factors that contribute to women's wealth gap are systemic, we've got to be aware of the role each of us plays. If we raise our awareness of ways we've been contributing to our financial challenges, we can do what Kerry Hannon suggests, and take control of our money.

Here are a few changes you can begin to make right now:

- **Be bolder in your career choices.** While women have made considerable progress moving into fields that pay more, such as law, medicine, and banking, we still often gravitate to career paths that have traditionally paid less, such as teaching, public relations, retail, and administrative and support roles, to name a few. If you're considering switching careers, explore the possibilities available in higher-paying industries such as technology, engineering, and management consulting, as well as law, medicine, and banking. While not all women have these options, based on their education, skills, and other realities, too many of us talk ourselves out of these career choices without carefully considering them.

- **Confront and transform the double whammy of lack of knowledge and lack of confidence.** These two are closely linked and have been shown to be what can hold us back from financial investing. According to a recent Fidelity survey, only 33 percent of women feel confident in their ability to make investment decisions. Even worse is our lack of knowledge: a mere 14 percent of women say they know a lot about saving and investing.[15] And there is a direct link between gaining knowledge and feeling confident. To boost your knowledge—and, in the process, your financial confidence—subscribe to reputable financial newsletters or blogs, listen to podcasts by financial experts, and take advantage of online courses, often available at no cost or low cost. Be wary of financial advice on social media unless it is from a vetted financial expert. This is a tangible step we must take.

- **Proactively involve yourself with family financial decision-making.** Many women in mixed-gender relationships delegate investing and large financial decision-making to their male spouse/partner. It's a stereotypical division of labor according to gender roles that our parents and grandparents often followed, so it feels comfortable. On top of that, we're busy, and financial decision-making can feel like one more thing to deal with when our plates are overflowing with "to-dos." Combined with that lack of confidence and education surrounding money matters, this causes many women to defer to their male partners when it comes to investing—even many executive women. I used to let Ken handle all the major investment decisions until the early 2000s, when Age Wave started researching women and money. That's when I started to see the costs—both financial and emotional—of not being a full participant in my own financial future. Now I'm investing in all kinds of new ways, from stocks to real estate and even a little venture capital (more on both of these later in the chapter).

- **Break the taboo on meaningful financial conversations.** In the same Age Wave study I referred to earlier, "Women and Money: Beyond the Bottom Line," we found that 61 percent of women would rather talk about their own death than money. We don't like to talk about, read about, or compare strategies for money and investing, and it holds us back. Ric Edelman confirmed this:

> There is still a powerful social taboo that keeps us from talking about money. These days, people talk about sex, drugs, politics, religion, but they still don't talk about money. Parents don't talk about it with their children. It's not taught in schools. Most employers don't help their workers with it. And so, people grow up financially illiterate, and yet they're faced with financial decisions, literally, on a daily basis.

It's time to bust this taboo, for our own sake and that of the generation we're raising. You can start by talking about your spending, saving, and investing strategies and questions with your friends and loved ones, including your kids. You can take it further and swap financial information and resources with those you trust most. I know it can be scary, but openly sharing will help remove some of the confusion and embarrassment. It can also encourage financial literacy for everyone involved, especially your kids.

- **Create and communicate financial boundaries with loved ones.** Forty-three percent of women have tapped their retirement savings to lend or give money to family members in need.[16] It's noble, and may legitimately feel like it's the only caring choice, but it also imperils our own future and, just as importantly, our lifelong financial peace of mind. A huge fear for women is being a burden on our children and grandchildren, which is a scenario that becomes a lot more likely when we deplete our savings.

- **Move past your fears and take financial action.** Most women, no matter how well-off financially, have a fear of outliving their money and ending up destitute. Viewed through a historical context, it's understandable—not so long ago, if a woman wasn't married, or if her husband died, she had few financial resources available to her because women couldn't inherit property and there were few professions open to women. The roots of this fear go deep, and this particular brand of anxiety can either inspire you to get yourself on a better financial footing or negatively influence you to be too conservative with the money you do have and hide it in your mattress, stick your head in the sand, and miss powerful opportunities to grow your nest egg. The answer is to take action now. "Just do something," as Lorna Sabbia, head of retirement and personal wealth solutions at Bank of America Merrill Lynch, told me. This may mean creating a budget for the first time (I did this recently, and it was eye-opening), tracking your monthly spending habits, starting an automatic withdrawal from your checking account into an investment account (even $50 or $100 a month is helpful), or seeking financial advice from a financial professional you can trust.

- **Own your financial agency.** Many of us women have inherited beliefs and attitudes toward money from our mothers and grandmothers, who did not have a lot of agency over their financial lives. We're blazing a new path, so let's embrace it.

- **Be a financial role model.** Forty-five percent of women say they do not have a financial role model.[17] This is a loss because role models inspire us with their example, provide motivation when we need to dig deep, and offer a road map for achieving our goals. Let's change this now. Choose to be a financial role model for your children, your grandchildren, and millions of young women who want and need to feel more financially empowered. Talk about your goals, fears, and choices with them. Let's show them the way!

KNOWLEDGE BRINGS CONFIDENCE: A BASIC PRIMER OF FINANCIAL TERMS

Saving and investing are full of jargon and acronyms, which can be a real barrier to having the knowledge and confidence to invest in your future. It's much easier to trust your own ability to make investing decisions when you understand some of the basic financial language, so let's dive into a few basics.

- **Saving vs. investing.** Saving is putting money aside that is earmarked for use in the near- to mid-term; savings are not meant for covering immediate expenses. Savings are held in an easily accessible (liquid) form, whether that's in a savings account, money market account, certificate of deposit, or coffee can hidden in the back of a closet. Please don't keep the majority of your savings in cash, as you'll miss out on the magic of compounding. Sure, keep enough to cover a couple of weeks in case the grid goes down. Otherwise, put it somewhere it can grow.

Investing, on the other hand, is using your money to become a stakeholder in an asset that will potentially grow over time. That could mean buying stocks, bonds, real estate, art, or crypto, or giving money to an early-stage business in return for a portion of future profits, equity, or proceeds.

A key distinction between the two is that saving is setting money aside for specific shorter-term needs, like a new roof, a vacation, or in case of an emergency, while investing is meant to build long-term funds for your future self. You need both.

- **Compound interest.** Compounding returns is what happens when the interest or returns you earn in your savings, money market, and investment accounts start earning interest on themselves, along with the interest earned on the principal or original amount invested. That means if you invest $1,000 today in an account that pays either interest, such as a savings or money market account, or dividends, such as stocks or mutual funds, and you choose to automatically reinvest those dividends and don't withdraw those funds, in forty years that $1,000 will have grown exponentially—with the biggest gains coming in the last ten years. To reap the benefits of compounding, once you start investing, stay invested.

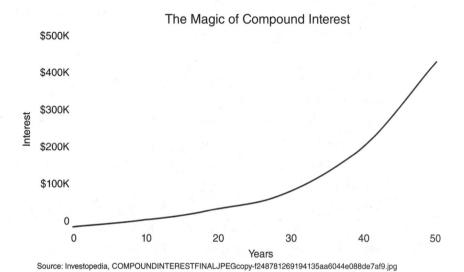

Source: Investopedia, COMPOUNDINTERESTFINALJPEGcopy-f248781269194135aa6044e088de7af9.jpg

Keep in mind that compounding interest in the form of credit card fees is something you want to avoid or, at the very least, minimize. That's when any credit card balances you have incur interest, and then you start being charged interest on the interest you owe, as well as on the original price of whatever you bought.

Compounding *returns* are what you want to take full advantage of; compounding *fees* are what you want to eliminate. So, as important as it is to save and invest your money, you also need to pay down your high-interest debt (like credit cards or lines of credit) as quickly as you can and make it a practice to pay your full balance each month.

- **Common acronyms.** Reading financial articles can feel like wading through a bowl of alphabet soup. Some of the most important acronyms you need to understand are:
  - ◦ **401(k).** This is a defined-contribution program or an employer-sponsored retirement investment account, designed to make it easy to invest by automatically diverting a portion of each paycheck. Funds you put into a 401(k) aren't taxed until you withdraw them, so they help reduce your tax burden in the present while providing a bigger base for growth. And many employers match at least a portion of the funds, which is essentially free money. Make sure to at least put enough money in your 401(k) to earn the matching funds, and ideally divert as much of your paycheck as you can into it. There are limits to how much you can invest in a 401(k); as I write this, that limit is $22,500 annually.
  - ◦ **Individual Retirement Account (IRA).** Similar to a 401(k), an IRA is designed to help you save for retirement using pre-tax dollars and is available to anyone. You don't need to go through your employer, as with a 401(k). If you withdraw funds from an IRA before age 59½, not only will it cost you the loss of those funds gaining compound interest, but you will have to pay a penalty. IRAs are offered through nearly all the major financial services companies and therefore have

a lot more investment options than a 401(k); you can also comparison-shop for the institution that has the lowest fees with the highest historical returns. It is possible to have both a 401(k) and an IRA.

- ◦ **529 plan, to pay for education:** These accounts are designed to help you save for college, for a child, a grandchild, or even yourself. The money in these accounts has minimal impact on the amount of financial aid you or your child is eligible for and may have tax advantages, depending on your state.

- ◦ **Health Savings Account (HSA)**—This account lets you set aside money for healthcare expenses with pre-tax money. The major drawback to these plans is that you must also have a high-deductible health plan (HDHP), which is an insurance plan that generally only covers preventive services before the deductible kicks in. If you have a typical PPO or HMO health plan, you can't open an HSA. But if you have an HDHP, an HSA is a great way to make your healthcare dollars go further while also reducing your tax bill.

While of course there are more terms and strategies to learn, this small handful is enough to get you on your way. "The best advice I can give to women is to just jump in and get started. Don't wait to become a seasoned expert," Sabbia advises. "Women tend to want to do all their due diligence before they begin, but you'll only gain more confidence by doing."

No matter what age you are when you're reading this, it's not too late to start rewriting the outcome of your money story—especially when you get help from a trusted advisor.

FINDING A FINANCIAL GUIDE WHO'S RIGHT FOR YOU

Even with all the obstacles in our way, the number of women who either earn more than their male spouse/partner or earn about the same has tripled since the 1970s.[18] We're starting to come into our own on the asset or wealth front, too. According to a 2020 McKinsey report, "women are the next wave of growth in wealth management," collectively poised to be managing a total of $30 trillion in assets by the mid-2020s.[19]

Not surprisingly, the financial services industry has taken notice. Lorna Sabbia told me, "Women are a part of the market that is growing in leaps and bounds. They make some of the most important financial decisions for themselves and their families, whether it's around paying down debt, or making healthcare decisions, or investing, and that purchasing power cannot be ignored."

Let's keep in mind that financial decision-making is no easy task for anyone. It's really not a do-it-yourself project. Even once you gain financial knowledge and confidence, it's helpful to have guidance and direction from a financial expert you can trust.

There are generally three levels of financial advice available. Yes, there are variations on the theme, including firms like Ellevest that are focused on women clients exclusively, but knowing about these three levels will help you match your needs and assets with the right level of advice.

- **Robo-advisors.** This is the newest form of financial advice, and it's best for people who are just starting out and have limited assets, as it's the least expensive option with no personal touch. Robo-advisors use computer algorithms to create and manage an investment portfolio for you based on your answers to an online questionnaire. They generally have very low or no account minimums, but only a few offer the service of getting questions answered by a real person. Search online for "best robo-advisors."
- **Self-directed financial advice.** This is where you make all the investment decisions yourself but use an online platform for investing. It is a hybrid, middle-of-the-road option—your investments are managed by an algorithm, so costs are lower. However, you also have access to an actual human to answer your specific questions and get guidance on other parts of your

financial life, such as saving for college or retirement. Meetings are usually virtual rather than face-to-face. Search online for "best online financial advisors."

- **Traditional financial advisors.** If you are looking for a higher level of service, where your investments are chosen by a real person or team of people, this is for you. If you think you need to be rich to have a financial advisor, think again. Ric Edelman told me, "These days, there's really no excuse for people not to get started with a financial advisor. Increasingly, there are human organizations that will work with you even if you don't have a lot of money. It's become far more inclusionary." This is great news. I recommend finding a financial advisor who is fiduciary. That means they have to put their client's needs ahead of their own.

Penny Pennington, managing partner at Edward Jones Investments, offers this advice to women on how to get the most value out of a relationship with a financial advisor: "Ask a lot of questions. Financial advisors are here to help, and they're happy to answer every question you have. There's no reason to be shy about it. Don't end the conversation with unanswered questions still in your head. And if you think of more afterwards, set up more time with your financial advisor to keep talking."

You'll know you've found a potentially good fit when you feel completely comfortable asking your advisor all your "dumb" questions, so don't hold back in your initial meetings. Hannon also suggests that many women may want to work with female financial advisors. She told me about meeting her husband's male financial advisor when they were first married: "When I met with him, he never even looked at me." This is a story I've heard a million times and experienced myself, too. According to Hannon, "he just talked to my husband, and here I was writing for *Forbes* magazine at the time! I actually knew a fair amount about finances and money. We walked out of the meeting, and I said, 'I'm not giving him a cent.'" She found a female advisor she's crazy about and has never looked back—and eventually her husband started to work with this woman, too.

No matter what type of advisor you choose, just remember that you are the ultimate decision-maker. "It's your money. Which means you need to participate. It's not out of sight, out of mind," Hannon said.

HOW MUCH YOU NEED TO SAVE
FOR RETIREMENT AND LONGEVITY

While financial advisors can be extremely helpful, you need to help them help you by defining your goals. One huge question that most people don't know the answer to is how much money they'll need once they're retired and living on a fixed or limited income. This is complicated by not being able to know how long you might live. Luckily, there is a basic formula that can take a lot of the guesswork out of retirement planning. This is not an exact science but will help you create some financial peace of mind. Some of the things to keep in mind:

- **Assume that you'll live to a hundred.** It's just what we all need to do in this era of longer lifespans.
- **Figure out your projected annual expenses.** You need an educated guess of how much money you'll need each year after you retire. The best way to make that guess is to outline what you're currently spending. While that may change in retirement, don't worry too much about that right now. This is not a fun exercise, but it's definitely worthwhile and necessary if you want to know how much you will need annually during years you may not be working or working part- or flex-time. If you're anything like me, you'll avoid doing this not-so-fun step. However, when Ken and I finally sat down to calculate how much we spend every year, it created a huge sense of relief.
- **Start with this basic formula.** Once you have your annual expenses estimated, multiply that number by the number of years you won't

be working. That equals the approximate amount of money you'll need for retirement.

- **Account for inflation.** You need to assume a 2.8 percent inflation rate annually. Add that into the formula by using an online inflation calculator, such as the one on BLS.gov (the website for the U.S. Bureau of Labor and Statistics), to see how much your current annual expenses will be in the future.[20]
- **Course-correct every few years.** The answer this formula provides may change over time, maybe growing larger or smaller. You will likely need to revisit this process every few years.

THE HEALTH/WEALTH EQUATION

Since finances are intricately tied to health in a variety of ways, health can be a powerful motivator for getting your financial house in order. The Aspen Institute has reported that health is intimately tied to both income and wealth—across all economic classes, people who earn less or have less wealth are less healthy than those who earn more or have more wealth.[21]

While the word *wealth* may derive from *well-being*, well-being often requires that you spend money. The holistic recipe we've talked about throughout the book entails spending more on higher-quality foods, exercise, supplements, healthcare providers, and health insurance. Though Medicare covers some of your healthcare expenses once you are age sixty-five or disabled, there can still be a lot of out-of-pocket health-related expenses.

However, consider this money as much an investment as an expense, because when you spend on your health, especially preventive measures, you improve the odds that your healthspan will align more closely with your lifespan. Plus, the money you spend on protecting your health can even save you money in the long term by reducing your healthcare costs in the future.

Katy Votava, an expert on personal healthcare costs, Medicare, and long-term care and also president and founder of Goodcare.com, told me, "Healthcare costs can derail an entire financial retirement plan. They are a basic financial responsibility, particularly if you're doing any kind of retirement planning."

Some cold, hard numbers can also be motivating, so let's start with $194,000. That's how much more the average woman spends out of pocket on healthcare in retirement than the average man, thanks to our longer lives, earlier retirement, and increased susceptibility to chronic diseases that require more healthcare.[22]

When it comes to health and wealth, it's a chicken-and-egg situation—you need money to promote health, but figuring out how much money you need and how you're going to pay for it can be stressful, which then harms your health. What's the way forward, then? Raise your awareness of the obstacles, make a plan to deal with them, and get the professional support and advice you need to choose and stick to that plan.

Medicare Explained

Many women eagerly await the day they turn sixty-five and can be covered by Medicare, thinking that means all their healthcare costs will be free. Medicare is not free. What it *is* is incredibly confusing and complicated. Simply put, Medicare is a U.S. federal health insurance program for those of us sixty-five and older, plus younger adults with disabilities. It consists of several parts, which I will attempt to explain below.

- **Part A.** This is the free part of Medicare. It pays for hospital and some skilled nursing facility stays, hospice care, most lab tests, and some, but not all, home healthcare.
- **Part B.** This part of Medicare helps to pay for doctor visits, outpatient care, some preventive services, and even some medical supplies. You need to pay the federal government for this coverage—how much depends on your yearly income—and there may be a penalty if you don't sign up for Part B when you turn sixty-five.

- **Part C.** This is where you might get really confused. This is also called Medicare Advantage or Medigap insurance and is meant to supplement Medicare Parts A and B. It's purchased by you (the insured) from private insurance companies. Part C is optional…kind of. It fills the gaps in Medicare coverage, paying deductibles, co-payments, and co-insurance payments. To add to the confusion, there are different Medigap plans offering different kinds of coverage, which is why you really need a Medicare consultant or a knowledgeable financial professional to help you figure out what you need.
- **Part D.** This also is paid by you and helps to pay for prescription drugs. Part D, too, is offered by private insurance companies. "Even if you aren't currently on any medications, you're better off having a basic prescription drug plan that you can modify down the road, because if you're suddenly in need of a medication that's $5,000 a month, that can really ruin your retirement savings," Katy Votava said. The private insurance plan you choose will greatly depend on which prescription drugs you take. These plans are definitely not one-size-fits-all and not only cover different drugs, but also have different costs.

When it comes to Medicare Part C and Medicare Part D, you need to comparison-shop. Votava told me, "Up to 95 percent of people in Medicare are overpaying out of pocket because they didn't select a plan that adequately covers their needs—perhaps their provider is out of network or their medications aren't fully covered." Again, I highly recommend doing some homework and then finding a great Medicare consultant to help navigate you to the right choice. A Medicare consultant doesn't have to be pricey. Instead, they may end up saving you considerable money in the form of healthcare expenses not covered by your Medicare plan. My cousin recently turned sixty-five and was getting overwhelmed by trying to navigate her Medicare enrollment. She did a quick search for a Medicare consultant online, found one she could meet with virtually, and found the right coverage for her specific healthcare needs in about an hour. The total cost? $200.

UNPACKING LONG-TERM CARE

While the very phrase "long-term care" makes you think you might need coverage that lasts a lifetime, Votava tells me that, on average, most people need long-term care for less than three years. You either need to set aside sufficient funds for this in advance or get long-term care insurance coverage just for that length of time so you can have peace of mind without totally breaking the bank. She's a fan of what's known as a "short, fat policy," which means it provides a lot of coverage for a relatively short amount of time. If you end up needing care for longer than three years, Votava says, the costs are so high, even with long-term care insurance, it is likely you will become eligible for Medicaid around the same time as your long-term care coverage runs out.

It's also important to have conversations with your loved ones, when everyone is healthy, about your wishes should you become ill, and their willingness to chip in with care. You also want to have your health-related legal documents in order, such as a living will, power of attorney, and healthcare proxies.

By choosing your insurance carefully, doing some thinking in advance, and tending to all the ingredients in your ageless aging holistic recipe, "you're going to be in the best position you can be in," Votava said. Unfortunately, there really isn't a "go-to" source for researching long-term care insurance options. You start by talking to a financial advisor or insurance agent who is knowledgeable about long-term care policies. However, advisors or agents sometimes only sell one brand of insurance. In that case, you should get quotes from multiple advisors/agents. You can also go to longtermcare.gov for more background information on long-term care planning and the website of the National Association of Insurance Commissioners (naic.org) and search for their "Consumer's Guide to Long-Term Care Insurance."[23]

— ◆ —

HOW EACH OF US CAN BE A PHILANTHROPIST

Lynne Twist introduced me to an idea I had never really thought about. She described three ways she believes women think about money that determine how generous we are with ourselves, our family and friends, and the world at large.

The first mindset she labeled "scarcity," which is the pervasive idea that there are not enough resources to go around. She explained that, yes, there are many people who don't have enough money to take care of themselves and their family and experience true scarcity, and we need to help those people whenever we can. But many of us have our basic needs covered, yet are driven by the fear of not having enough. The scarcity mentality leads to the idea that we always need more. As a result, we never feel like we have enough money, no matter how much we might have.

The second mindset she described is "sufficiency." That's the state of knowing on a deep level that you have enough, and that ultimately all your needs—and at least some of your wants—are covered. It's a feeling of appreciation for what you have and not a longing for what you don't.

The third mindset she described is one of "abundance," which flows from sufficiency but goes further. It's what she described as "having so much enough-ness that it overflows so that you are able to cover all your expenses and also share genuinely and generously with others."

Abundance is the source of philanthropy, which may seem like it's just about giving money away but is actually more expansive than that. The etymology of the word *philanthropy* means "love of humankind." That means each of us can be a philanthropist, regardless of the size of our bank account. In fact, each of us should be a philanthropist, because "there is no one who doesn't have a role to play in bringing forth the more beautiful world that we all know is possible," Twist said.

While philanthropy often does entail giving money, you can also be a philanthropist by giving of your time, love, attention, effort, energy, and service. One thing philanthropy does require is a shift in mindset away from scarcity and toward abundance. Twist describes it as a shift from fear to love. "When you know you have enough, it's your chance and your privilege to roll up your sleeves and help make things work more effectively," she explained.

Chances are there's already a cause or a group of people you are involved in. If so, you are on the right track and keep going! If you've felt like you don't have enough money to give back, challenge yourself to root out the thoughts, beliefs, and ideas that tell you if you give to others there won't be enough for you. There are always ways to give back. And when you do, you stand to gain just as much as the people or causes you are helping. "When you know that you're seeking to make a difference with your money, your time, and your life, you feel joyful and fulfilled. You feel more alive," Twist told me. And that feeds your well-being, which, remember, is the true meaning of wealth.

CUTTING-EDGE APPROACHES TO STRENGTHEN YOUR WEALTH/HEALTH CONNECTION

- **Impact investing.** "Impact investing has been around for a while, but now it's really hitting its stride," says Trish Costello, founder and CEO of Portfolia, a collaborative equity investment platform designed specifically for women to invest in the companies they most want to see in the marketplace. "For a long time, the reality and the expectation were that if you invested for impact, you'd have to give up good returns. But the truth is, today, you don't have to give up anything in terms of return for impact." According to the Global Impact Investing Network, 88 percent of impact investors say the strategy either is in line with (68 percent) or exceeds (20 percent) their financial expectations.[24]

  Women and younger adults are leading the charge on impact investing, because, Costello said, "women take a more holistic view. If you're putting a product out that is bad for the world in some way but could make you a lot of money, the majority of women will say, 'I don't want that.'" If we're going to be living as long as we are, and because we are so naturally attuned to taking care of the generations that come after us, impact investing is a way to infuse your financial strategy with a broader, longer-term meaning and purpose.

Many robo-advisors and online financial advisors as well as traditional financial advisory firms have impact investing options. There are also certain funds, known as ESG (environment, social, and governance) funds, that you can invest in directly through an online brokerage account. If you want to choose specific companies to invest in to create your own impact portfolio, request their impact or sustainability report so that you can research their intended goals and their quantifiable impacts.

- **Venture investing through membership.** Venture capital is investing in early-stage businesses when their potential for growth and providing returns is at its highest—although it's important to point out that this is also when they have the highest likelihood of failure, so venture investing can be risky. Venture capital (VC) has traditionally only been available to the very wealthy, often with a minimum initial investment of $100,000 and sometimes $1 million. Not anymore. An emerging trend in VC is to pool resources from a group of investors so individuals can gain access to the VC world, with all its potential risks and rewards, for a much lower initial investment. Many of these groups allow you to combine impact investing with VC investing by enabling you to invest in companies that are seeking to create solutions to issues you care about. For example, Energea (energea.com) enables you to invest in renewable energy start-ups around the world for as little as $100, while VentureSouth (venturesouth .vc) lets you invest in your local community of entrepreneurs if you live in the South. I am a lead partner for the Active Aging and Longevity 2 fund at Portfolia (portfolia.co), the venture membership for women that Trish Costello founded, which offers access to multiple funds organized around various subjects such as climate change, longevity, and women-owned companies. Portfolia lets you really learn the VC ropes, attending pitch meetings and voting on which companies the fund will invest in, and requires a minimum investment of $10,000.

- **Crypto investing.** Cryptocurrency, or crypto for short, is a digital form of currency that is encrypted (so it can't be counterfeited) and is stored on multiple computer networks, so it doesn't require a central bank to store it or regulate it. Because crypto is still an emerging technology, it is very volatile. While its future is uncertain, many people believe it is also a technology that is likely to play a progressively bigger role in our financial system and so will likely become more valuable over time.

  When I asked Ric Edelman if women should invest in crypto, he didn't hesitate. "Absolutely," he said, not least because "more than 90 percent who own crypto are men," likely because women are less likely to engage in risky investments. He recommends investing just 1 percent of your net worth in crypto—not enough to hurt when it goes through its inevitable crashes on the path to stability, but also enough to help build wealth over the long term if it comes into its own.

- **"Paycheck for life" insurance products.** While annuities have been around for a long time, the financial industry has reinvented them for the twenty-first century, making annuities more targeted toward providing steady income for long-lived adults. The majority of women say their number-one financial goal is to live long with more financial security and peace of mind.[25] These "paychecks for life" annuities are financial products that are designed to provide just that. They allow you to invest an amount up front; it will then start paying a regular monthly amount at a date in the future that you decide on. Those payments will continue as long as you are alive, whether you live to 85, 95, or 105. While annuities are not a new concept, what is relatively new is that they typically no longer have the high fees they once did, which eroded their financial benefit. You can invest any amount that makes sense to you, based on how much money you think you will need every month to make up the gap between whatever income you'll be receiving (from Social Security, a pension, and whatever other investment income you may have) and what you think you'll need to cover your expenses. Plus you can start with a small annuity now and then bump it up later once you have a clearer idea of your expenses and your lifespan and healthspan. Talk with your financial advisor or insurance consultant about it or visit the Alliance for Lifetime Income website (protectedincome.org).

THE WEALTH/HEALTH CONNECTION: WHERE TO BEGIN

If you do one thing: Max out your 401(k) if you're employed or your SEP IRA if you're self-employed

Invest heavily in your future self and enjoy the magic of compounding by investing each year regularly and withdrawing only if there's a real emergency and you have no other alternative, as withdrawing the funds before you hit age 59½ costs you in fees and a 10 percent penalty, plus that money then won't be able to continue to grow. This is admittedly easier if you receive a regular paycheck and have a 401(k), as it's a decision you only need to make once and then a portion of each paycheck will be automatically added to your 401(k). If you are self-employed, you'll have to write a check or initiate a transfer each time you want to contribute to your SEP. Get around this hurdle by building a habit of taking 15 percent of the amount each time you are paid and sending it directly to your SEP IRA. If you take the money out immediately, you have significantly less opportunity to miss it.

If you're a beginner: Gain financial literacy

You don't need to become a financial expert, but it's wise to learn the jargon and some basic understanding of budgeting, saving, and investing. Much of this information is readily available online: all the major brokerage firms have educational content that you don't have to be a client to access, as do apps such as Mint and Acorns and websites such as Investopedia, NerdWallet, and Motley Fool. In the real world, many community centers, libraries, and community colleges offer financial literacy classes, and financial advisors worth their salt can be a valuable source of education as well. Just like traveling to any foreign country, once you speak even a little bit of the language, you'll start to feel a lot more at home, your fear will ease, and your confidence will rise.

If you're ready to take it to the next level: Close that wealth gap

Start to think like a breadwinner: proactively negotiate for raises, perks, and promotions; prioritize investing; and start thinking about what you already own or can create that will pay you directly, without wholly relying on a paycheck for your income. Use each paycheck to help you invest in your future self, and shift your mindset from scarcity (focusing on paying the bills) to sufficiency (diversifying your income and investments so that you trust yourself to always have enough), and then even to abundance (thinking of yourself as a philanthropist).

AGELESS AGING HACKS TO STRENGTHEN YOUR WEALTH/HEALTH CONNECTION

Reduce or eliminate your debt

Besides investing in your future self, one of the best financial steps you can take is to pay down your debt, especially high-interest debt such as credit card debt.

Know it's never too late to get started investing

If you're in your fifties, you could still have forty-plus years for your investments to grow. So don't be discouraged, but take action now.

Schedule a regular money talk with your partner/spouse

Money (along with sex) is one of the top two things couples fight about. Keep the air clear between the two of you by scheduling a regular money date. Ken and I just did this around our budget, which loomed large for months with both of us avoiding the conversation. However, once we did it, the meeting took all of forty-five minutes and made both of us feel better emotionally, more in alignment with each other, and more financially confident. Besides budgeting, you might want to discuss your estate plan, what big expenses you have coming up, and how you can invest more.

Start a money circle

Enroll a handful of friends to sit down together every month and talk about money and investing in your future selves. It can be a social event, whether you go out for drinks or have a potluck dinner at someone's house. You can also invite a guest speaker from your local college or a financial firm to educate the group on a particular subject like impact investing or lifetime annuities. This can benefit anyone, but especially solo agers. "You just want to talk to somebody about your finances, and knock ideas around with," Hannon explains. Maybe it's sharing things you've recently read in an article or a book or heard on a podcast. While yes, it's good to learn from experts, it's also extremely helpful to learn from each other in a supportive environment where no question is too "dumb" and no idea is too "crazy."

We all need safe spaces to learn, so be that for each other. You could take it one step further and turn your money circle into an investment club, where you collectively discuss potential investments—stocks, bonds, mutual funds, annuities, et cetera—and gain the benefit of having more minds thinking through the pros and cons. Or you can join an investment club for women that already exists, such as InvestingFixx (investingfixx.com) from women's financial experts Jean Chatzky (the financial ambassador for AARP, the financial editor for the NBC show *Today* for twenty-five years, and a multiple-bestselling author) and Karen Finerman (CEO of the Metropolitan Capital Advisors hedge fund in New York City and author of the bestselling book *Finerman's Rules: Secrets I'd Only Tell My Daughters About Business and Life*).

Talk to your financial advisor alone and together with your partner/spouse

Oftentimes couples will share a financial advisor. However, Hannon recommends making sure that you talk to that advisor not only with your partner/spouse but on your own sometimes, too. "Even though I love and trust my husband, I feel more comfortable asking questions and free to talk about my financial life without him in the meeting," she told me.

Hire a Medicare consultant

Now that you can see how confusing and overwhelming Medicare can be, find a knowledgeable consultant who knows the exact questions to ask and what information you need, and who can analyze your options and provide you with some solid choices. It will save you hours of worry and possibly a lot of money. A good place to start looking is your state health insurance assistance program (start at shiphelp.org). Because Medicare coverages can vary by state, you can also search online for "Medicare consultant" and add your state name.

Make course corrections again and again

You can make course corrections that create more financial peace of mind and real assets for your longer life throughout your life. For example, in an Age Wave/Edward Jones 2023 study, "Resilient Choices: Tradeoffs, Adjustments and Course Corrections to Thrive in Retirement," we used an example of a fifty-year-old divorced woman who decided to develop a financial strategy to catch up on her retirement savings. She finds a higher-paying job, with a salary of $10,000 more per year and with a better employer match of 6 percent on her retirement savings. She also finds a housemate to share costs. She buys a more economical car, and she may also decide to start a weekend side gig that pays an extra $7,500 a year that she can invest into her IRA.

By taking these steps, not only did she increase her financial confidence and prospects to thrive in her longer life, but from a practical standpoint, she is saving $17,000 per year and earning $10,000 more per year. She's also now able to contribute $27,000 more per year over the next fifteen years to her investments. The bottom line? Her asset balance at the age of sixty-five increases from $237,000 to $992,000—or $1,173,000 with the side gig. This example shows you what's possible even at age fifty. So get out of paralysis and make a move. Your future self will be grateful you did, both because you'll have more financial security and peace of mind, and because your health tends to improve as your wealth increases.

Next Steps

◆

CREATE YOUR AGELESS AGING ACTION PLAN

As important as it is to learn new information and increase your knowledge, it's only when you implement that learning by taking action that you can create true change. I know that I've given you a long list of things you can do to extend your healthspan, grow your current and future peace of mind, and help you make the most of your longevity bonus, and that having a long list can be overwhelming. Keep in mind that you can't do it all, but you have to do something. It's about finding the right mix of strategies that work for you, and continuing to build on your healthy habits. Each change you make gives you more momentum, energy, and motivation.

As you chart your course, keep in mind these two recommendations:

- **Remember, when it comes to making changes, one size does not fit all.** As Dr. Stephen Kopecky advised in Chapter 1, making one or two small changes can feel very doable and create a lot of noticeable improvements over time. However, if you're facing a serious health situation, you might need to make more and bigger changes all at once. Or you may simply be motivated to jump in with both feet now, an approach that has its upside.

As Dr. Dean Ornish told me, "Making big changes all at once is a pound of cure as opposed to an ounce of prevention." You can even move between these two approaches, ramping up when your motivation is high, and dialing it back when you need a little time to settle into your new healthy habits. Of course, you want to be realistic and honest with yourself about how many changes you can implement—or handle—at once but be bold in believing in your ability to make changes that will help you feel more energized and fulfilled.

- **Let joy lead the way.** Both Dr. Ornish and Chungliang Al Huang counseled finding the joy of living and feeling better. Move your ultimate goal away from fear—preventing something bad from happening, like a heart attack or stroke years down the road—to the joy of living and feeling better now and well into the future.

To help you evaluate your options and choose where you'll start, here's a checklist that recaps recommendations from each chapter of the book. Winnow down your options by checking off the hacks you're not interested in or are already doing. Then decide which tools you're ready to start using, and prioritize your efforts there. In fact, when you've gone through the complete list, get out your highlighter and highlight the three, four, or five strategies that are a top priority for you so that there's no confusion about what you should get to work on.

Refer back to this list periodically to help you stay in touch with the changes you want to make, and to find inspiration for new strategies you want to implement as you continue on your ageless aging journey.

— ◆ —

Chapter 1: Sipping from the Fountain of Youthfulness

Take the Ageless Aging Self-Assessment

Choose one accelerant to stop doing

Choose one decelerant to start doing

Chapter 2: Embracing the Upsides of Long Life

Talk about your own—and others'—ageist assumptions

Foster an intergenerational friendship

Become a mentern

Host or participate in a Generations Over Dinner

Listen to recently released music

Visualize your ideal ageless aging journey

Chapter 3: Charting Your Path

Write down five things you know you want for yourself as you age
(such as a strong friend network or a hobby that engages your mind and body)

Choose a starting point

Make a plan

Write down your goals

Start practicing the art of "plussing"

Write down in your calendar the ageless aging ingredients you're committing to

Consider an NAC supplement or prioritizing cysteine-rich foods

Chapter 4: Fitness 2.0, the Silver Bullet

Identify at least one additional type of fitness you'll try

Incorporate high-intensity intervals into your workout

Choose a strategy to improve your posture

Choose a strategy to interrupt your sitting

Identify at least one cutting-edge fitness option on page 95 that is right for you now

Make mornings your regular workout time

Spend three minutes a day moving quickly

Set up your home for more movement

Already doing	Not interested	Ready to start doing	Ready to take to the next level
_____	_____	_____	_____
_____	_____	_____	_____
_____	_____	_____	_____
_____	_____	_____	_____
_____	_____	_____	_____
_____	_____	_____	_____
_____	_____	_____	_____
_____	_____	_____	_____
_____	_____	_____	_____
_____	_____	_____	_____
_____	_____	_____	_____
_____	_____	_____	_____
_____	_____	_____	_____
_____	_____	_____	_____
_____	_____	_____	_____
_____	_____	_____	_____
_____	_____	_____	_____
_____	_____	_____	_____
_____	_____	_____	_____
_____	_____	_____	_____
_____	_____	_____	_____
_____	_____	_____	_____
_____	_____	_____	_____
_____	_____	_____	_____

(continues)

Try isometric contractions

Add a little manual labor back into your day

Chapter 5: Food Is Fuel, Food Is Medicine, Food Is Pleasure

Identify your diet-related goals

Eat five different-colored foods per day

Eat more fish and less red meat

Swap out unhealthy fats for healthy ones

Get the junk food (refined sweets and ultra-processed foods) out of your pantry

Go twelve to thirteen hours after dinner without eating

Stop eating three hours before bedtime

Drink half your body weight in ounces of water each day

Wean yourself off sugar, especially in your morning beverage

Try a mega-beverage

Stick to no alcohol or just one alcoholic beverage a day

Consider whether a longer fast, or fasting-mimicking diet, is right for you

Evaluate the cutting-edge nutrition options on
page 132 to determine if one is right for you now

Save money and boost health with frozen organic vegetables and fruits

Use the EWG's Dirty Dozen list to choose which produce you need to buy organic

When you need to drink bottled water, opt for Fiji, Gerolsteiner, or Volvic

Invest in extra-virgin olive oil

Make or buy bone broth

Chapter 6: The Magic of Sleep

Use the SATED questionnaire to assess your sleep quality

Choose two things from "Your Daytime To-Do
List to Sleep Better at Night" on page 148

Train yourself to get out of bed and do something soothing
when you wake up in the middle of the night

Evaluate the cutting-edge sleep options on pages 156–158
to determine if one is right for you now

Choose and stick to a consistent wake time

Already doing	Not interested	Ready to start doing	Ready to take to the next level
————	————	————	————
————	————	————	————
————	————	————	————
————	————	————	————
————	————	————	————
————	————	————	————
————	————	————	————
————	————	————	————
————	————	————	————
————	————	————	————
————	————	————	————
————	————	————	————
————	————	————	————
————	————	————	————
————	————	————	————
————	————	————	————
————	————	————	————
————	————	————	————
————	————	————	————
————	————	————	————
————	————	————	————
————	————	————	————
————	————	————	————
————	————	————	————

(continues)

Expose yourself to daylight first thing in the morning

Write out your list of top worries during the day

Have more orgasms

Try mouth tape

Unwind with NSDR or yoga nidra

Add two minutes of breathing exercises to your bedtime routine

Chapter 7: You Are the CEO of Your Own Healthcare

Find a primary care doctor you trust

Prepare for doctor's visits and write your questions down in advance

Ask questions and advocate for yourself

Educate yourself from reputable sources

Invest your money in your health, wellness, and healthcare

Stay current on your appointments and screenings

Evaluate the pelvic health options on page 171
to determine if one is right for you now

Evaluate the cutting-edge pain options on page 172
to determine if one is right for you now

Decide which diagnostic tests make sense for you and discuss with your doctor

Evaluate the cutting-edge health options on page 180
to determine if one is right for you now

Get to know your community pharmacist

Look into a concierge medical practice if that makes sense for you

Consider an NAD+ precursor in supplement form

Consider nitric oxide supplements

Consider a CoQ10 supplement if you take statins

Chapter 8: Hormones Are Your Frenemies

Fill out the Menopause Rating Scale on pages 196–198

Evaluate the cutting-edge hormone options on pages 211–212
to determine if one is right for you now

Schedule a DEXA scan if you've never had one, or talk to your doctor about
when to have your next one if it's been more than a year

Already doing	Not interested	Ready to start doing	Ready to take to the next level
_____	_____	_____	_____
_____	_____	_____	_____
_____	_____	_____	_____
_____	_____	_____	_____
_____	_____	_____	_____
_____	_____	_____	_____
_____	_____	_____	_____
_____	_____	_____	_____
_____	_____	_____	_____
_____	_____	_____	_____
_____	_____	_____	_____
_____	_____	_____	_____
_____	_____	_____	_____
_____	_____	_____	_____
_____	_____	_____	_____
_____	_____	_____	_____
_____	_____	_____	_____
_____	_____	_____	_____
_____	_____	_____	_____
_____	_____	_____	_____
_____	_____	_____	_____

(continues)

Find a doctor certified in menopausal medicine

Evaluate the hormone hacks on pages 215–217
to determine if one might be right for you now

Chapter 9: Your Beautiful Mind

Consider whether brain imaging is a good choice for you to determine
if you have the plaques or tangles associated with dementia

Try to figure things out for yourself before asking for help

Commit to learning a new skill

Do more math in your head before opening up the calculator on your phone

If you have high blood pressure, treat it

Have your hearing evaluated, and wear hearing aids if you need them

Stop smoking (hypnosis may help)

Lose a little bit of weight if that's right for you

(Finally) try meditation

Reframe negative experiences with positive thoughts

Eat fermented foods and/or take probiotics

Review the brain-supportive supplements on pages 230–231
to determine if one is right for you now

Evaluate the cutting-edge brain health options on pages 233–237
to determine if one is right for you now

Exercise with friends, while doing things
that require focus, or outside at least once a week

Practice gratitude

Inhale and exhale for a count of four each whenever you feel stressed

Drink warm water with lemon first thing in the a.m.

Stay hydrated throughout the day

Commit to never skipping a morning or evening brushing, flossing, and tongue scraping

Invest in Alzheimer's research

Chapter 10: Purpose and Connection

Inventory your relationships and how often you see and connect with people

Do big or tiny acts of kindness every day

Already doing	Not interested	Ready to start doing	Ready to take to the next level
_____	_____	_____	_____
_____	_____	_____	_____
_____	_____	_____	_____
_____	_____	_____	_____
_____	_____	_____	_____
_____	_____	_____	_____
_____	_____	_____	_____
_____	_____	_____	_____
_____	_____	_____	_____
_____	_____	_____	_____
_____	_____	_____	_____
_____	_____	_____	_____
_____	_____	_____	_____
_____	_____	_____	_____
_____	_____	_____	_____
_____	_____	_____	_____
_____	_____	_____	_____
_____	_____	_____	_____
_____	_____	_____	_____
_____	_____	_____	_____
_____	_____	_____	_____
_____	_____	_____	_____

(continues)

Prioritize continuing to make new friends by joining a group, religious community, or organization (or adopt a dog)

Evaluate the cutting-edge approaches to fostering purpose and connection on page 259 to determine if one is right for you now

Volunteer at least one hour a week

Decide if there is a friendship or relationship you need to end or restructure because it's weighing you down or holding you back

Reach out to a new potential friend or someone you've lost contact with to reestablish the connection

Get a manicure, massage, or other hands-on treatment with no guilt

Plan a trip with your grandchildren

Chapter 11: The Wealth-Health Connection

Ask for a raise, other benefits, and perks

Actively seek out financial knowledge, via books, websites, and podcasts

Actively participate in your family's financial tasks and decisions

Start a money circle to talk about financial topics and tools

Get started investing, or up your investments if you've already started

Find a financial advisor that's a good fit for you, if you don't already have one

Calculate how much money you're likely to need in retirement

If you're sixty-five or older, find a Medicare consultant to help you get the health coverage you need

Talk to your loved ones about your wants and needs for long-term care

Get your healthcare proxy, living will, and power of attorney in order

Find ways to be a philanthropist

Evaluate the cutting-edge approaches to finances on pages 286–289 to determine if one is right for you now

Max out your 401(lk) or SEP IRA contributions

Prioritize paying your high-interest debt (such as credit card balances)

Schedule a regular money talk with your spouse or partner

Talk to your financial advisor together with your spouse and alone

Already doing	Not interested	Ready to start doing	Ready to take to the next level

ACKNOWLEDGMENTS

From Maddy Dychtwald:

Books, like most creative endeavors, are team efforts. I was lucky enough to have a first-rate team to both help turn my idea into this special book and support me for years in the process. My heartfelt thanks to all those wonderful people who have contributed to this process.

My husband, Ken, for being both my soulmate and my workmate, a hard duo to pull off. You shower me with love, and provide emotional resilience, knowledge, and a critical eye when needed. I'm so glad we're on this life adventure together!

My fantastic kids, Casey and Zak, whom I love so deeply. You both inspire me to be a better person and have taught me a thing or two about manifesting dreams.

My incredible daughter-in-law, FeyFey, whose encouragement and cheerleading made me want to keep going.

My close circle of family, Richard, Linda, Joel, Patty and Lucas, David, Michelle, Annie, Jonah and Jacob Verkh-Kent, as well as Alan Dychtwald and his partner, Aleli Haar.

My writing partner extraordinaire, Kate Hanley, whose know-how, intelligence, insights, enthusiasm, and strong writing chops made for a great partnership.

My Age Wave family, Elyse Pellman (best buddy in and out of work), Robyn Reynolds, Katy Flick Terveer, Bob Morrison, Thi Truong, Neil Steinberg, Luke Van Meter, Samantha Cebers,

Ruth Bercovich, and Jason Welshonse, for being my extended family and for their commitment to digging deep into aging and longevity through our research, graphics, plussing of ideas, support, and enthusiasm so critical to bringing this book to life.

Amy Garcia, whose knowledge, wisdom, thoughtful insights, and editorial sculpting were instrumental in streamlining my message.

Jane von Mehren at Aevitas Creative Management, for being not only an amazing agent (yes, you are!), but also a true partner in creating the bones of this book. And a shout-out to Will Lippincott at Aevitas, who knew Jane and I would make a great team. Thanks for the introduction.

Daniela Rapp, senior acquisitions editor at Mayo Clinic Press, for believing in my vision, giving me support and guidance along the way, and taking this journey with me to help women in their quest for a more ageless aging.

The Harris Poll team, including Humphrey Taylor and David Krane.

The best-of-the-best committed and brilliant researchers, scientists, doctors, experts, and friends who so generously gave me their time to be interviewed to share their wisdom, knowledge, experience, expertise, and candid insights for this book: Ashton Applewhite, Katy Bowman, Dr. Jim Bramson, Dr. Laura Carstensen, Dr. Gaël Chételat, Nikki Chrysostomou, Dr. Hassy Cohen, Meryl Comer, Chip Conley, Trish Costello, Helen Dennis, Joan Ditzion, Carolyn Drury, Ric and Jean Edelman, Dr. Kara Fitzgerald, Marc Freedman, Linda Fried, Dr. Jennifer Garrison, Sara Zeff Geber, Lisa Genova, Dr. Felice Gersh, Dana Griffin, Kerry Hannon, Dr. Kelli Harding, Chungliang "Al" Huang, Arianna Huffington, Nancy Katz, Dr. James Kirkland, Kristin Kirkpatrick, Dr. Stephen Kopecky, Dr. Daniel Kraft, Dr. Carol Kuhle, Dr. Suzanne LeBlang, Carolee Lee, Dr. Valter Longo, Dr. Beth McDougall, Colin

Milner, Rita Moreno, Anne and Dean Ornish, Dr. Pam Peeke, Penny Pennington, Dr. Andrea Pfeifer, Dr. Christina Pham, Dr. Aric Prather, Dr. Krista Ramonas, Lorna Sabbia, Ann Seclow, Dr. Suzanne Steinbaum, Nadia Tuma-Weldon, Lynne Twist, Katy Votava, and Dr. Phyllis Zee. Words don't begin to express my deep gratitude and respect.

Special thanks to Dr. Christina Y. Chen, assistant professor of medicine at Mayo Clinic, for her additional expertise and generous dedication of her time in reviewing the manuscript.

Others who contributed their wise words, ideas, and personal stories, including Dr. Neel Anand, Jennifer Barrett, Dr. Elizabeth Blackburn, Quin Bommelje, Dr. Gavin Britz, Dan Buettner, Stephen Covey, Christopher Exley, Susan Felicissimo, Tim Ferriss, Jane Fonda, Ying-Hui Fu, Cassie Holmes, Dr. Andrew Huberman, Denise Kaufman, Mary Ellen Klee, Becca Levy, Joan McDonald, Marc Middleton, Helen Mirren, Lisa Mosconi, Dr. Vivek Murthy, Dr. Maiken Nedergaard, Dolly Parton, Michael Pollan, Carla Prado, Louis Ptacek, Mary Rawles, Melody-Rose, Dr. John Rowe, Alan Rozanski, Dr. Mark I. Ryder, DeEtte Sauer, Ann Seclow, Dr. David Sinclair, Dr. Carolyn Swenson, Dr. Robert Waldinger, Oprah Winfrey, and Wendy Wood.

My early readers, who helped sculpt the final book, including Sandie Dorman, Zak Dychtwald, Amy Garcia, and my Age Wave family.

Friends and colleagues, who make my life richer and more meaningful: Cindi Fox; Bodil Arlander; Cecilia Arradaza; Sonia Arrison; Jayme Canton; Becca Derrough; Sandie and Kenny Dorman; JoeMax Floyd; Mary Furlong; Ahri, Jay, Izzy, and Sofia Golden; Stacy Haller; Nancy, Danny, Justin, and Liza Katz; Michael and Leslie Krasny; Sabina Loetscher; Nancy Lyn; Anna Nakayasu; Manthi Nguyun; Stuart Pellman; Chantell Preston; Trisha Stewart; Elizabeth Torres; Matthew and Jessica Upchurch; George Vradenburg; Nancy and Gordon Wheeler; and Dave, Robin, and Grace Zaboski.

Celene Santos and Jennifer Brennan, who are instrumental in making my life work.

From Kate Hanley:

My heartfelt thanks to Maddy Dychtwald for being an inspiring and gracious collaborator, to Daniela Rapp for her insightful guidance, to Madeleine Morel for having my back, to my girlfriends for tolerating my proselytizing about all the information and strategies I learned about while working on this book, and to Scott, Lillian, and Teddy for being my everything.

NOTES

CHAPTER 1

1. Viña, J., Borrás, C., Gambini, J., Sastre, J., & Pallardó, F. V. (2005). Why females live longer than males: Control of longevity by sex hormones. *Science of Aging Knowledge Environment: SAGE KE, 2005*(23), pe17. https://doi .org/10.1126/sageke.2005.23.pe17; Global Health Observatory, World Health Organization. (2020, December 4). "Healthy Life Expectancy (HALE) at birth (years)." https://www.who.int/data/gho/data/indicators/indicator-details/GHO /gho-ghe-hale-healthy-life-expectancy-at-age-60.
2. Barrett, A. E., & von Rohr, C. (2008). Gendered perceptions of aging: An examination of college students. *International Journal of Aging & Human Development, 67*(4), 359–386. https://doi.org/10.2190/AG.67.4.d.
3. Levy, B. R., Slade, M. D., Kunkel, S. R., & Kasl, S. V. (2002). Longevity increased by positive self-perceptions of aging. *Journal of Personality and Social Psychology, 83*(2), 261–270. https://doi.org/10.1037 //0022-3514.83.2.261.
4. Levy, B. R., Zonderman, A. B., Slade, M. D., & Ferrucci, L. (2009). Age stereotypes held earlier in life predict cardiovascular events in later life. *Psychological Science, 20*(3), 296–298. https://doi.org/10.1111 /j.1467-9280.2009.02298.x.
5. Levy, B. R., Chung, P. H., Slade, M. D., Van Ness, P. H., & Pietrzak, R. H. (2019). Active coping shields against negative aging self-stereotypes contributing to psychiatric conditions. *Social Science & Medicine, 228*, 25–29. https://doi.org/10.1016/j.socscimed.2019.02.035.
6. Levy, B. R., Slade, M. D., Murphy, T. E., & Gill, T. M. (2012). Association between positive age stereotypes and recovery from disability in older persons. *JAMA, 308*(19), 1972–1973. https://doi.org/10.1001/jama.2012.14541.
7. Levy, B. R., Slade, M. D., Pietrzak, R. H., & Ferrucci, L. (2018). Positive age beliefs protect against dementia even among elders with high-risk gene. *PLoS ONE, 13*(2), article e0191004. https://doi.org/10.1371/journal .pone.0191004.
8. Kwak, S., Kim, H., Chey, J., & Youm, Y. (2018). Feeling how old I am: Subjective age is associated with estimated brain age. *Frontiers in Aging Neuroscience, 10*, 168. https://doi.org/10.3389/fnagi.2018.00168.

CHAPTER 2

1. Edward Jones and Age Wave. (2022). Longevity and the new journey of

retirement. https://www.edwardjones.com/us-en/market-news-insights
/retirement/new-retirement/longevity.

2. Blanchflower, D. G., & Oswald, A. J. (2008). Is well-being U-shaped over the life cycle? *Social Science & Medicine, 66*(8), 1733–1749. https://doi .org/10.1016/j.socscimed.2008.01.030; Wunder, C., Wiencierz A., Schwarze, J., & Küchenhoff, H. (2013). Well-being over the life span: Semiparametric evidence from British and German longitudinal data. *Review of Economics and Statistics, 95*(1), 154–167. http://www.jstor.org /stable/23355657.

3. Zenger, J., & Folkman, J. (2016). How age and gender affect self-improvement. *Harvard Business Review.* https://hbr.org/2016/01/how-age-and -gender-affect-self-improvement.

4. Abrams, M. (2022, October 3). Andie MacDowell rocks gray hair on Paris Fashion Week runway. *New York Post.* https://pagesix.com/2022/10/03/andie -macdowell-rocks-gray-hair-on-paris-fashion-week-runway/.

5. Costello, R. B., Elin, R. J., Rosanoff, A., Wallace, T. C., Guerrero-Romero, F., Hruby, A., Lutsey, P. L., Nielsen, F. H., Rodriguez-Moran, M., Song, Y., & Van Horn, L. V. (2016). Perspective: The case for an evidence-based reference interval for serum magnesium: The time has come. *Advances in Nutrition, 7*(6), 977–993. https://doi.org/10.3945/an.116.012765.

6. Kalie, A. M. (2015). "Music was better back then": When do we stop keeping up with popular music? Skynet & Ebert. https://skynetandebert.com/2015/04 /22/music-was-better-back-then-when-do-we-stop-keeping-up-with-popular -music/.

7. Bloodworth, A. (2021). How to get back into new music—and why it's so good for you. *Huffington Post.* https://www.huffingtonpost.co.uk/entry /new-music-listening-over-30-new-music-psychology_uk_5fff21bac5b656719 88b22e9.

CHAPTER 3

1. Anguah, K. O., Syed-Abdul, M. M., Hu, Q., Jacome-Sosa, M., Heimowitz, C., Cox, V., & Parks, E. J. (2019). Changes in food cravings and eating behavior after a dietary carbohydrate restriction intervention trial. *Nutrients, 12*(1), 52. https://doi.org/10.3390/nu12010052.

2. Lally, P., Van Jaarsveld, C H. M., Potts, H. W. W., & Wardle, J. (2010). How are habits formed: Modelling habit formation in the real world. *European Journal of Social Psychology, 40*(6), 998–1009. doi: 10.1002/ejsp.674.

3. Horsch, C., Spruit, S., Lancee, J., Van Eijk, R., Beun, R. J., Neerincx, M., & Brinkman, W.-P. (2017). Reminders make people adhere better to a self-help sleep intervention. *Health and Technology, 7,* 173–188.

4. Zalachoras, I., Ramos-Fernández, E., Hollis, F., Trovo, L., Rodrigues, J., Strasser, A., Zanoletti, O., Steiner, P., Preitner, N., Xin, L., Astori, S., & Sandi, S. (2022). Glutathione in the nucleus accumbens regulates motivation to exert reward-incentivized effort. *eLife, 11,* e77791. https://doi.org/10.7554 /eLife.77791.

5. McCarty, M. F., & DiNicolantonio, J. J. (2015). An increased need for dietary cysteine in support of glutathione synthesis may underlie the increased risk for mortality associated with low protein intake in the elderly. *Age, 37*(5), 96.

CHAPTER 4

1. Barrès, R., Yan, J., Egan, B., Treebak, J. T., Rasmussen, M., Fritz, T., Caidahl, K., Krook, A., O'Gorman, D. J., & Zierath, J. R. (2012). Acute exercise remodels promoter methylation in human skeletal muscle. *Cell Metabolism*, *15*(3), 405–411. https://doi.org/10.1016/j.cmet.2012.01.001.

2. Moore, S. C., Lee, I. M., Weiderpass, E., Campbell, P. T., Sampson, J. N., Kitahara, C. M., Keadle, S. K., Arem, H., Berrington de Gonzalez, A., Hartge, P., Adami, H. O., Blair, C. K., Borch, K. B., Boyd, E., Check, D. P., Fournier, A., Freedman, N. D., Gunter, M., Johannson, M., Khaw, K. T., et al. (2016). Association of leisure-time physical activity with risk of 26 types of cancer in 1.44 million adults. *JAMA Internal Medicine*, *176*(6), 816–825. https://jamanetwork.com/journals/jamainternalmedicine/fullarticle/2521826.

3. Hooker, S. P., Diaz, K. M., Blair, S. N., et al. (2022). Association of accelerometer-measured sedentary time and physical activity with risk of stroke among US adults. *JAMA Network Open, 5*(6), e2215385. doi:10.1001/jamanetworkopen.2022.15385.

4. Smith, A. D., Crippa, A., Woodcock, J., & Brage, S. (2016). Physical activity and incident type 2 diabetes mellitus: A systematic review and dose-response meta-analysis of prospective cohort studies. *Diabetologia*, *59*(12), 2527–2545. https://doi.org/10.1007/s00125-016-4079-0.

5. Lee, D. H., Rezende, L. F. M., Joh, H.-K., Keum, N., Ferrari, G., Rey-Lopez, J. P., Rimm, E. B., Tabung, F. K., & Giovannucci, E. L. (2022). Long-term leisure-time physical activity intensity and all-cause and cause-specific mortality: A prospective cohort of US adults. *Circulation, 146*(7), 523–534. https://doi.org/10.1161/CIRCULATIONAHA.121.058162.

6. Turner, C. H., & Robling, A. G. (2004). Exercise as an anabolic stimulus for bone. *Current Pharmaceutical Design*, *10*(21), 2629–2641. https://doi.org/10.2174/1381612043383755.

7. Alzheimer's disease: Can exercise prevent memory loss? (May 12, 2021). Mayo Clinic. https://www.mayoclinic.org/diseases-conditions/alzheimers-disease/expert-answers/alzheimers-disease/faq-20057881; Physical exercise and dementia (n.d.). Alzheimer's Society. https://www.alzheimers.org.uk/about-dementia/risk-factors-and-prevention/physical-exercise.

8. Harvard Health Publishing. Exercise and Fitness. https://www.health.harvard.edu/topics/exercise-and-fitness, accessed December 9, 2022.

9. Master, H., Annis, J., Huang, S., Beckman, J. A., Ratsimbazafy, F., Marginean, K., Carroll, R., Natarajan, K., Harrell, F. E., Roden, D. M., Harris, P., & Brittain, E. L. (2022). Association of step counts over time with the risk of chronic disease in the All of Us Research Program. *Nature Medicine*, *28*(11), 2301–2308. https://doi.org/10.1038/s41591-022-02012-w; Paluch, A. E., Bajpai, S., Bassett, D. R., Carnethon, M. R., Ekelund, U., Evenson, K. R., Galuska, D. A., Jefferis, B. J., Kraus, W. E., Lee, I. M., Matthews, C. E., Omura, J. D., Patel, A. V., Pieper, C. F., Rees-Punia, E., Dallmeier, D., Klenk, J., Whincup, P. H., Dooley, E. E., Pettee Gabriel, K., et al. Steps for Health Collaborative (2022). Daily steps and all-cause mortality: A meta-analysis of 15 international cohorts. *The Lancet Public Health*, *7*(3), e219–e228. https://doi.org/10.1016/S2468-2667(21)00302

-9; Paluch A. E., Gabriel, K. P., Fulton, J. E., et al. (2021). Steps per day and all-cause mortality in middle-aged adults in the Coronary Artery Risk Development in Young Adults Study. *JAMA Network Open, 4*(9), e2124516. doi:10.1001/jamanetworkopen.2021.24516.

10. Robinson, M. M., Dasari, S., Konopka, A. R., Johnson, M. L., Manjunatha, S., Esponda, R. R., Carter, R. E., Lanza, I. R., & Nair, K. S. (2017). Enhanced protein translation underlies improved metabolic and physical adaptations to different exercise training modes in young and old humans. *Cell Metabolism, 25*(3), 581–592. https://doi.org/10.1016/j.cmet.2017.02.009.

11. Moreau, D., & Chou, E. (2019). The acute effect of high-intensity exercise on executive function: A meta-analysis. *Perspectives on Psychological Science: A Journal of the Association for Psychological Science, 14*(5), 734–764. https://doi.org/10.1177/1745691619850568.

12. Maillard, F., Pereira, B., & Boisseau, N. (2018). Effect of high-intensity interval training on total, abdominal and visceral fat mass: A meta-analysis. *Sports Medicine, 48*(2), 269–288. https://doi.org/10.1007/s40279-017-0807-y.

13. Trapp, E. G., Chisholm, D. J., Freund, J., & Boutcher, S. H. (2008). The effects of high-intensity intermittent exercise training on fat loss and fasting insulin levels of young women. *International Journal of Obesity, 32*(4), 684–691. https://doi.org/10.1038/sj.ijo.0803781.

14. Caan, B. J., Cespedes Feliciano, E. M., Prado, C. M., Alexeeff, S., Kroenke, C. H., Bradshaw, P., Quesenberry, C. P., et al. (2018). Association of muscle and adiposity measured by computed tomography with survival in patients with nonmetastatic breast cancer. *JAMA Oncology, 4*(6), 798–804.

15. Prado, C. M., Purcell, S. A., Alish, C., Pereira, S. L., Deutz, N. E., Heyland, D. K., Goodpaster, B. H., Tappenden, K. A., & Heymsfield, S. B. (2018). Implications of low muscle mass across the continuum of care: A narrative review. *Annals of Medicine, 50*(8), 675–693. https://doi.org/10.1080/07853890.2018.1511918.

16. Melov, S., Tarnopolsky, M. A., Beckman, K., Felkey, K., & Hubbard, A. (2007). Resistance exercise reverses aging in human skeletal muscle. *PloS ONE, 2*(5), e465. https://doi.org/10.1371/journal.pone.0000465.

17. National Center for Complementary and Integrative Health. (2022, March). Tai chi: What you need to know. https://www.nccih.nih.gov/health/tai-chi-what-you-need-to-know.

18. Araujo, C. G., de Souza e Silva, C. G., Laukkanen, J. A., et al. (2022). Successful 10-second one-legged stance performance predicts survival in middle-aged and older individuals. *British Journal of Sports Medicine, 56*, 975–980.

19. Andersen, C. H., Shiffer, E., & Lam, J. (2022), Do posture correctors actually help you stand straighter? Experts weigh in. *Women's Health*. https://www.womenshealthmag.com/health/a28385621/best-posture-correctors/.

20. Wipfli, B., Landers, D., Nagoshi, C., & Ringenbach, S. (2011). An examination of serotonin and psychological variables in the relationship between exercise and mental health. *Scandinavian Journal of Medicine & Science in Sports, 21*, 474–481. https://doi.org/10.1111/j.1600-0838.2009.01049.x.

21. Patel, A. V., Bernstein, L., Deka, A., Feigelson, H. S., Campbell, P. T., Gapstur, S. M., Colditz, G. A., & Thun, M. J. (2010). Leisure time spent sitting in relation to total mortality in a prospective cohort of US adults. *American Journal of Epidemiology*, 172(4), 419–429. https://pubmed.ncbi.nlm.nih.gov/20650954/.

22. Haller, J. M., Roberts, D. E., & Freedson, P. S. (2006). Increasing energy expenditure during sedentary activity. *Medicine & Science in Sports & Exercise*, 38(5), S367; Rizzato, A., Marcolin, G., & Paoli, A. (2022). Non-exercise activity thermogenesis in the workplace: The office is on fire. *Frontiers in Public Health*, 10, 1024856. https://doi.org/10.3389/fpubh.2022.1024856.

23. Larsen, R. N., Kingwell, B. A., Sethi, P., Cerin, E., Owen, N., & Dunstan, D. W. (2014). Breaking up prolonged sitting reduces resting blood pressure in overweight/obese adults. *Nutrition, Metabolism, and Cardiovascular Diseases*, 24(9), 976–982. https://doi.org/10.1016/j.numecd.2014.04.011; Brocklebank, L. A., Andrews, R. C., Page, A., Falconer, C. L., Leary, S., & Cooper, A. (2017). The acute effects of breaking up seated office work with standing or light-intensity walking on interstitial glucose concentration: A randomized crossover trial. *Journal of Physical Activity & Health*, 14(8), 617–625. https://doi.org/10.1123/jpah.2016-0366.

24. Buffey, A. J., Herring, M. P., Langley, C. K., Donnelly, A. E., & Carson, B. P. (2022). The acute effects of interrupting prolonged sitting time in adults with standing and light-intensity walking on biomarkers of cardiometabolic health in adults: A systematic review and meta-analysis. *Sports Medicine*, 52(8), 1765–1787. https://doi.org/10.1007/s40279-022-01649-4.

25. Ekblom-Bak, E., Ekblom, B., Vikström, M., de Faire, U., & Hellénius, M. L. (2014). The importance of non-exercise physical activity for cardiovascular health and longevity. *British Journal of Sports Medicine*, 48(3), 233–238. https://doi.org/10.1136/bjsports-2012-092038.

26. Villablanca, P. A., Alegria, J. R., Mookadam, F., Holmes, D. R., Jr., Wright, R. S., & Levine, J. A. (2015). Nonexercise activity thermogenesis in obesity management. *Mayo Clinic Proceedings*, 90(4), 509–519. https://doi.org/10.1016/j.mayocp.2015.02.001.

27. Jaquish, J. (2013). Multiple-of-bodyweight axial bone loading using novel exercise intervention with and without bisphosphonate use for osteogenic adaptation. *Osteoporosis International*, 24(4), s594–s595; Hunte, B., Jaquish, J., & Huck, C. (2015). Axial bone osteogenic loading-type resistance therapy showing BMD and functional bone performance musculoskeletal adaptation over 24 weeks with postmenopausal female subjects. *Journal of Osteoporosis & Physical Activity*, 3(146), 2; Huck, C., & Jaquish, J. (2015). Functional bone performance measurements and adaptations using novel self-applied bone loading exercise apparatus. *Osteoporosis International*, 26(1), s391–s392.

28. Pano-Rodriguez, A., Beltran-Garrido, J. V., Hernandez-Gonzalez, V., & Reverter-Masia, J. (2020). Effects of whole-body electromyostimulation on physical fitness in postmenopausal women: A randomized controlled trial. *Sensors*, 20(5), 1482. https://doi.org/10.3390/s20051482.

29. Albalak, G., Stijntjes, M., Van Bodegom, D., Jukema, J. W., Atsma, D. E., Van Heemst, D., & Noordam, R. (2022). Setting your clock: Associations between timing of objective physical activity and cardiovascular disease risk in

the general population. *European Journal of Preventive Cardiology*, zwac239. https://doi.org/10.1093/eurjpc/zwac239; Aird, T. P., Davies, R. W., & Carson, B. P. (2018). Effects of fasted vs fed-state exercise on performance and post-exercise metabolism: A systematic review and meta-analysis. *Scandinavian Journal of Medicine & Science in Sports, 28*(5), 1476–1493. https://doi .org/10.1111/sms.13054.

30. Rasmussen, L. J. H., Caspi, A., Ambler, A., Broadbent, J. M., Cohen, H. J., d'Arbeloff, T., Elliott, M., Hancox, R. J., Harrington, H., Hogan, S., Houts, R., Ireland, D., Knodt, A. R., Meredith-Jones, K., Morey, M. C., Morrison, L., Poulton, R., Ramrakha, S., Richmond-Rakerd, L., Sison, M. L., et al. (2019). Association of neurocognitive and physical function with gait speed in midlife. *JAMA Network Open, 2*(10), e1913123. https://doi.org/10.1001 /jamanetworkopen.2019.13123.

31. Stamatakis, E., Ahmadi, M. N., Gill, J. M. R., Thøgersen-Ntoumani, C., Gibala, M. J., Doherty, A., & Hamer, M. (2022). Association of wearable device-measured vigorous intermittent lifestyle physical activity with mortality. *Nature Medicine, 28*, 2521–2529. 10.1038/s41591-022-02100-x.

CHAPTER 5

1. Belman, O. (2018, February 2). What to know about fasting, aging, the "longevity diet," and when you should eat. USC News. https://news.usc.edu /135551/fasting-aging-dieting-and-when-you-should-eat-valter-longo/.

2. Sun, Y., Liu, B., Snetselaar, L. G., Wallace, R. B., Caan, B. J., Rohan, T. E., Neuhouser, M. L., et al. (2019). Association of normal-weight central obesity with all-cause and cause-specific mortality among postmenopausal women. *JAMA Network Open, 2*(7), e197337.

3. Hibi, M., et al. (2018). Efficacy of tea catechin-rich beverages to reduce abdominal adiposity and metabolic syndrome risks in obese and overweight subjects: A pooled analysis of 6 human trials. *Nutrition Research, 55*, 1–10. https://doi.org/10.1016/j.nutres.2018.03.012.

4. Stylianou, K. S., Fulgoni, V. L., & Jolliet, O. (2021). Small targeted dietary changes can yield substantial gains for human health and the environment. *Nature Food, 2*, 616–627. https://doi.org/10.1038/s43016-021-00343-4.

5. Mundi, M. (2022, May 5). What is intermittent fasting? Does it have health benefits? Mayo Clinic. https://www.mayoclinic.org/healthy-lifestyle/nutrition -and-healthy-eating/expert-answers/intermittent-fasting/faq-20441303.

6. Barnosky, A. R., Hoddy, K. K., Unterman, T. G., & Varady, K. A. (2014). Intermittent fasting vs daily calorie restriction for type 2 diabetes prevention: A review of human findings. *Translational Research: The Journal of Laboratory and Clinical Medicine, 164*(4), 302–311. https://doi.org/10.1016/j.trsl .2014.05.013.

7. Dmitrieva, N. I., Gagarin, A., Liu, D., Wu, C. O., & Boehm, M. (2023). Middle-age high normal serum sodium as a risk factor for accelerated biological aging, chronic diseases, and premature mortality. *EBioMedicine, 87*, 104404. https://doi.org/10.1016/j.ebiom.2022.104404.

8. Wei, M., Brandhorst, S., Shelehchi, M., Mirzaei, H., Cheng, C. W., Budniak, J., Groshen, S., Mack, W. J., Guen, E., Di Biase, S., Cohen, P., Morgan, T. E.,

Dorff, T., Hong, K., Michalsen, A., Laviano, A., & Longo, V. D. (2017). Fasting-mimicking diet and markers/risk factors for aging, diabetes, cancer, and cardiovascular disease. *Science Translational Medicine, 9*(377), eaai8700. https://doi.org/10.1126/scitranslmed.aai8700.

9. D'Andrea Meira, I., Romão, T. T., Pires do Prado, H. J., Krüger, L. T., Pires, M. E. P., & da Conceição, P. O. (2019). Ketogenic diet and epilepsy: What we know so far. *Frontiers in Neuroscience, 13*(5), https://doi.org/10.3389/fnins.2019.00005.

10. Weber, D. D., Aminzadeh-Gohari, S., Tulipan, J., Catalano, L., Feichtinger, R. G., & Kofler, B. (2020). Ketogenic diet in the treatment of cancer—where do we stand? *Molecular Metabolism, 33*, 102–121. https://doi.org/10.1016/j.molmet.2019.06.026.

11. Hersant, H., & Grossberg, G. (2022). The ketogenic diet and Alzheimer's disease. *Journal of Nutrition, Health & Aging, 26*(6), 606–614. https://doi.org/10.1007/s12603-022-1807-7.

12. National Heart, Lung, and Blood Institute. (2021, December 29). The science behind the DASH eating plan. https://www.nhlbi.nih.gov/education/dash/research.

13. Morris, M. C., Tangney, C. C., Wang, Y., Sacks, F. M., Bennett, D. A., & Aggarwal, N. T. (2015). MIND diet associated with reduced incidence of Alzheimer's disease. *Alzheimer's & Dementia: The Journal of the Alzheimer's Association, 11*(9), 1007–1014. https://doi.org/10.1016/j.jalz.2014.11.009; Hosking, D. E., Eramudugolla, R., Cherbuin, N., & Anstey, K. J. (2019). MIND not Mediterranean diet related to 12-year incidence of cognitive impairment in an Australian longitudinal cohort study. *Alzheimer's & Dementia: The Journal of the Alzheimer's Association, 15*(4), 581–589. https://doi.org/10.1016/j.jalz.2018.12.011.

14. Bellini, M., Tonarelli, S., Nagy, A. G., Pancetti, A., Costa, F., Ricchiuti, A., de Bortoli, N., Mosca, M., Marchi, S., & Rossi, A. (2020). Low FODMAP diet: Evidence, doubts, and hopes. *Nutrients, 12*(1), 148. https://doi.org/10.3390/nu12010148.

15. Konijeti, G. G., Kim, N., Lewis, J. D., Groven, S., Chandrasekaran, A., Grandhe, S., Diamant, C., Singh, E., Oliveira, G., Wang, X., Molparia, B., & Torkamani, A. (2017). Efficacy of the autoimmune protocol diet for inflammatory bowel disease. *Inflammatory Bowel Diseases, 23*(11), 2054–2060. https://doi.org/10.1097/MIB.0000000000001221; Abbott, R. D., Sadowski, A., & Alt, A. G. (2019). Efficacy of the autoimmune protocol diet as part of a multi-disciplinary, supported lifestyle intervention for Hashimoto's thyroiditis. *Cureus, 11*(4), e4556. https://doi.org/10.7759/cureus.4556.

16. Makovicky, P., Makovicky, P., Caja, F., Rimarova, K., Samasca, G., & Vannucci, L. (2020). Celiac disease and gluten-free diet: Past, present, and future. *Gastroenterology and Hepatology from Bed to Bench, 13*(1), 1–7.

17. Krysiak, R., Szkróbka, W., & Okopień, B. (2019). The effect of gluten-free diet on thyroid autoimmunity in drug-naïve women with Hashimoto's thyroiditis: A pilot study. *Experimental and Clinical Endocrinology & Diabetes: Official Journal, German Society of Endocrinology [and] German Diabetes Association, 127*(7), 417–422. https://doi.org/10.1055/a-0653-7108.

18. Estruch, R., Ros, E., Salas-Salvadó, J., Covas, M. I., Corella, D., Arós, F., Gómez-Gracia, E., Ruiz-Gutiérrez, V., Fiol, M., Lapetra, J., Lamuela-Raventos, R. M., Serra-Majem, L., Pintó, X., Basora, J., Muñoz, M. A., Sorlí, J. V., Martínez, J. A., Fitó, M., Gea, A., Hernán, M. A., et al. for the PREDIMED Study Investigators (2018). Primary prevention of cardiovascular disease with a Mediterranean diet supplemented with extra-virgin olive oil or nuts. *New England Journal of Medicine, 378*(25), e34. https://doi.org/10.1056/NEJMoa1800389.

CHAPTER 6

1. Bhaskar, S., Hemavathy, D., & Prasad, S. (2016). Prevalence of chronic insomnia in adult patients and its correlation with medical comorbidities. *Journal of Family Medicine and Primary Care, 5*(4), 780–784. doi:10.4103/2249-4863.201153.
2. Desmet, L., Thijs, T., Segers, A., Verbeke, K., & Depoortere, I. (2021). Chronodisruption by chronic jetlag impacts metabolic and gastrointestinal homeostasis in male mice. *Acta Physiologica, 233*(4), e13703. https://doi.org/10.1111/apha.13703; Thaiss, C. A., Zeevi, D., Levy, M., Zilberman-Schapira, G., Suez, J., Tengeler, A. C., Abramson, L., Katz, M. N., Korem, T., Zmora, N., Kuperman, Y., Biton, I., Gilad, S., Harmelin, A., Shapiro, H., Halpern, Z., Segal, E., & Elinav, E. (2014). Transkingdom control of microbiota diurnal oscillations promotes metabolic homeostasis. *Cell, 159*(3), 514–529. https://doi.org/10.1016/j.cell.2014.09.048.
3. Bermingham, K. M., Stensrud, S., Asnicar, F., Valdes, A. M., Franks, P. W., Wolf, J., Hadjigeorgiou, G., Davies, R., Spector, T. D., Segata, N., Berry, S. E., Hall, W. L. (2023). Exploring the relationship between social jetlag with gut microbial composition, diet and cardiometabolic health, in the ZOE PREDICT 1 cohort. *European Journal of Nutrition*. DOI: 10.1007/s00394-023-03204-x.
4. Johns Hopkins Medicine (n.d.). Depression and sleep. Retrieved March 13, 2023, from https://www.hopkinsmedicine.org/health/wellness-and-prevention/depression-and-sleep-understanding-the-connection.
5. Wu, Y., Song, L., Wang, X., Li, N., Zhan, S., Rong, P., Wang, Y., & Liu, A. (2022). Transcutaneous vagus nerve stimulation could improve the effective rate on the quality of sleep in the treatment of primary insomnia: A randomized control trial. *Brain Sciences, 12*(10), 1296.
6. Dhand, R., & Sohal, H. (2006). Good sleep, bad sleep! The role of daytime naps in healthy adults. *Current Opinion in Pulmonary Medicine, 12*(6), 379–382. doi:10.1097/01.mcp.0000245703.92311.d0.
7. Kräuchi, K., Cajochen, C., Werth, E., & Wirz-Justice, A. (1999). Warm feet promote the rapid onset of sleep. *Nature, 401*, 36–37. https://doi.org/10.1038/43366.
8. Mogavero, M. P., Cosentino, F. I. I., Lanuzza, B., Tripodi, M., Lanza, G., Aricò, D., DelRosso, L. M., Pizza, F., Plazzi, G., & Ferri, R. (2021). Increased serum prolactin and excessive daytime sleepiness: An attempt of proof-of-concept study. *Brain Sciences, 11*(12), 1574. https://doi.org/10.3390/brainsci11121574.

CHAPTER 7

1. Dawson, C. M. P., Abiola, A. O., Sullivan, A. M., Schwartz, A. W., & members of the GERI Team Research Group (2022). You can't be what you can't see: A systematic website review of Geriatrics Online-Visibility at US medical schools. *Journal of the American Geriatrics Society, 70*(10), 2996–3005. https://doi.org/10.1111/jgs.17997; Gurwitz, J. H. (2023). The paradoxical decline of geriatric medicine as a profession. *JAMA, 330*(8), 693–694. https://doi.org/10.1001/jama.2023.11110.

2. Swenson, C., & Malani, P. (November 1, 2018). Urinary incontinence: An inevitable part of aging? National Poll on Healthy Aging. https://www.healthyagingpoll.org/reports-more/report/urinary-incontinence-inevitable-part-aging.

3. Wu, J. M., et al. (2009). Forecasting the prevalence of pelvic floor disorders in U.S. Women: 2010 to 2050. *Obstetrics and Gynecology, 114*(6), 1278–1283. https://doi.org/10.1097/AOG.0b013e3181c2ce96; Luber, K. M., et al. (2001). The demographics of pelvic floor disorders: Current observations and future projections. *American Journal of Obstetrics and Gynecology, 184*(7), 1496–1503. https://doi.org/10.1067/mob.2001.114868.

4. Kiesel, L. (2017, October 9). Women and pain: Disparities in experience and treatment. *Harvard Health Blog.* https://www.health.harvard.edu/blog/women-and-pain-disparities-in-experience-and-treatment-2017100912562.

5. Ruau, D., et al. (2012). Sex differences in reported pain across 11,000 patients captured in electronic medical records. *Journal of Pain, 13*(3), 228–234. https://doi.org/10.1016/j.jpain.2011.11.002.

6. Tsagkaris, C., Papazoglou, A. S., Eleftheriades, A., Tsakopoulos, S., Alexiou, A., Gāman, M.-A., & Moysidis, D. V. (2022). Infrared radiation in the management of musculoskeletal conditions and chronic pain: A systematic review. *European Journal of Investigation in Health, Psychology and Education, 12*(3), 334–343. doi:10.3390/ejihpe12030024.

7. Argueta, D. A., et al. (2020). A balanced approach for cannabidiol use in chronic pain. *Frontiers in Pharmacology, 11*(561). https://doi.org/10.3389/fphar.2020.00561.

8. Verdin, E. (2015). NAD$^+$ in aging, metabolism, and neurodegeneration. *Science, 350*(6265), 1208–1213. https://doi.org/10.1126/science.aac4854.

9. Covarrubias, A. J., et al. (2021). NAD$^+$ metabolism and its roles in cellular processes during ageing. *Nature Reviews: Molecular Cell Biology, 22*(2), 119–141. https://doi.org/10.1038/s41580-020-00313-x.

10. Mills, K. F., et al. (2016). Long-term administration of nicotinamide mononucleotide mitigates age-associated physiological decline in mice. *Cell Metabolism, 24*(6), 795–806. https://doi.org/10.1016/j.cmet.2016.09.013; Fang, E. F., et al. (2019). Mitophagy inhibits amyloid-β and tau pathology and reverses cognitive deficits in models of Alzheimer's disease. *Nature Neuroscience, 22*(3), 401–412. https://doi.org/10.1038/s41593-018-0332-9.

11. Yi, L., et al. (2023). The efficacy and safety of β-nicotinamide mononucleotide (NMN) supplementation in healthy middle-aged adults: A randomized, multicenter, double-blind, placebo-controlled, parallel-group, dose-dependent clinical trial. *GeroScience, 45*(1), 29–43. https://doi.irg/10.1007/s11357-022-00705-1; Chini, C. C., Guerrico, A. M., Nin, V., Camacho-Pereira,

J., Escande, C., Barbosa, M. T., & Chini, E. N. (2014). Targeting of NAD metabolism in pancreatic cancer cells: Potential novel therapy for pancreatic tumors. *Clinical Cancer Research: An Official Journal of the American Association for Cancer Research, 20*(1), 120–130. https://doi.org/10.1158/1078-0432.CCR-13-0150.

CHAPTER 8

1. Cleveland Clinic (2022, December 29). Progesterone. https://my.clevelandclinic.org/health/body/24562-progesterone.
2. Bonafide Health, LLC (n.d.). The state of menopause. Retrieved from https://hellobonafide.com/pages/state-of-menopause on May 11, 2023.
3. Stampfer, M. J., Colditz, G. A., Willett, W. C., Manson, J. E., Rosner, B., Speizer, F. E., & Hennekens, C. H. (1991). Postmenopausal estrogen therapy and cardiovascular disease. Ten-year follow-up from the nurses' health study. *New England Journal of Medicine, 325*(11), 756–762. https://doi.org/10.1056.
4. Dominus, S. (2022, February 1). Women have been misled about menopause. *New York Times Magazine.* https://www.nytimes.com/2023/02/01/magazine/menopause-hot-flashes-hormone-therapy.html.
5. Rossouw, J. E., Manson, J. E., Kaunitz, A. M., & Anderson, G. L. (2013). Lessons learned from the Women's Health Initiative trials of menopausal hormone therapy. *Obstetrics and Gynecology, 121*(1), 172; Manson, J. E., Hsia, J., Johnson, K. C., Rossouw, J. E., Assaf, A. R., Lasser, N. L., Trevisan, M., et al. (2003). Estrogen plus progestin and the risk of coronary heart disease. *New England Journal of Medicine, 349*(6), 523–534; Manson, J. E., Chlebowski, R. T., Stefanick, M. L., Aragaki, A. K., Rossouw, J. E., Prentice, R. L., Anderson, G., et al. (2013). Menopausal hormone therapy and health outcomes during the intervention and extended poststopping phases of the Women's Health Initiative randomized trials. *JAMA, 310*(13), 1353–1368; Santen, R. J., Allred, D. C., Ardoin, S. P., Archer, D. F., Boyd, N., Braunstein, G. D., Burger, H. G., et al. (2010). Postmenopausal hormone therapy: An Endocrine Society scientific statement. *Journal of Clinical Endocrinology & Metabolism, 95*(7, supp. 1), s1–s66.
6. Mehta, J., Kling, J. M., & Manson, J. E. (2021). Risks, benefits, and treatment modalities of menopausal hormone therapy: Current concepts. *Frontiers in Endocrinology, 12*, 564781.
7. Miller, V. M., Naftolin, F., Asthana, S., Black, D. M., Brinton, E. A., Budoff, M. J., Cedars, M. I., Dowling, N. M., Gleason, C. E., Hodis, H. N., Jayachandran, M., Kantarci, K., Lobo, R. A., Manson, J. E., Pal, L., Santoro, N. F., Taylor, H. S., & Harman, S. M. (2019). The Kronos Early Estrogen Prevention Study (KEEPS): What have we learned? *Menopause, 26*(9), 1071–1084. https://doi.org/10.1097/GME.0000000000001326; Taylor, H. S., Tal, A., Pal, L., Li, F., Black, D. M., Brinton, E. A., Budoff, M. J., Cedars, M. I., Du, W., Hodis, H. N., Lobo, R. A., Manson, J. E., Merriam, G. R., Miller, V. M., Naftolin, F., Neal-Perry, G., Santoro, N. F., & Harman, S. M. (2017). Effects of oral vs transdermal estrogen therapy on sexual function in early postmenopause: Ancillary study of the Kronos Early Estrogen Prevention Study (KEEPS). *JAMA Internal Medicine, 177*(10), 1471–1479. https://doi.org/10.1001/jamainternmed.2017.3877; Hodis, H. N., Mack, W. J., Shoupe, D.,

Azen, S. P., Stanczyk, F. Z., Hwang-Levine, J., Budoff, M. J., & Henderson, V. W. (2014). Testing the menopausal hormone therapy timing hypothesis: The early versus late intervention trial with estradiol. *Circulation, 130*, A13283. https://www.ahajournals.org/doi/10.1161/circ.130.suppl_2.13283.

8. Song, Y., Li, S., Li, X., Chen, X., Wei, Z., Liu, Q., & Cheng, Y. (2020). The effect of estrogen replacement therapy on Alzheimer's disease and Parkinson's disease in postmenopausal women: A meta-analysis. *Frontiers in Neuroscience, 14*. https://www.frontiersin.org/articles/10.3389/fnins.202.

9. Palmisano, B. T., Zhu, L., & Stafford, J. M. (2017). Role of estrogens in the regulation of liver lipid metabolism. *Advances in Experimental Medicine and Biology, 1043*, 227–256. https://doi.org/10.1007/978-3-319-70178-3_12.

10. Camilleri, M. (2019). Leaky gut: Mechanisms, measurement and clinical implications in humans. *Gut, 68*(8), 1516–1526. https://doi.org/10.1136/gutjnl-2019-318427.

11. Kronzer, V. L., Bridges, S. L., Jr., & Davis, J. M., 3rd (2020). Why women have more autoimmune diseases than men: An evolutionary perspective. *Evolutionary Applications, 14*(3), 629–633. https://doi.org/10.1111/eva.13167.

12. Alemany, M. (2021). Estrogens and the regulation of glucose metabolism. *World Journal of Diabetes, 12*(10), 1622–1654. doi:10.4239/wjd.v12.i10.1622.

13. Moffat, S. D., An, Y., Resnick, S. M., Diamond, M. P., & Ferrucci, F. (2020). Longitudinal change in cortisol levels across the adult life span. *Journals of Gerontology: Series A, 75*(2), 394–400. https://doi.org/10.1093/gerona/gly279.

14. Yiallouris, A., et al. (2019). Adrenal aging and its implications on stress responsiveness in humans. *Frontiers in Endocrinology, 10*(54). doi:10.3389/fendo.2019.00054.

15. Mayo Clinic Staff (2021). DHEA. https://www.mayoclinic.org/drugs-supplements-dhea/art-20364199.

CHAPTER 9

1. Livingston, G., Sommerlad, A., Orgeta, V., Costafreda, S. G., Huntley, J., Ames, D., et al. (2017). Dementia prevention, intervention, and care. *Lancet, 390*(10113), 2673-2734. https://doi.org/10.1016/S0140-6736(17)31363-6.

2. Livingston, G., Huntley, J., Sommerlad, A., Ames, D., Ballard, C., Banerjee, S., Brayne, C., Burns, A., Cohen-Mansfield, J., Cooper, C., Costafreda, S. G., et al. (2020). Dementia prevention, intervention, and care: 2020 report of the Lancet Commission. *Lancet, 396*(10248), 413–446. https://doi.org/10.1016/S0140-6736(20)30367-6.

3. Jaslow, R. (2023, April 19). Scientists regenerate hair cells that enable hearing. Harvard Medical School. https://hms.harvard.edu/news/scientists-regenerate-hair-cells-enable-hearing.

4. Veronese, N., Facchini, S., Stubbs, B., et al. (2017). Weight loss is associated with improvements in cognitive function among overweight and obese people: A systematic review and meta-analysis. *Neuroscience & Biobehavioral Reviews, 72*, 87–94.

5. Gomes Gonçalves, N., Vidal Ferreira, N., Khandpur, N., et al. (2023). Association between consumption of ultraprocessed foods and

cognitive decline. *JAMA Neurology, 80*(2), 142–150. doi:10.1001/jamaneurol.2022.4397.

6. Mosconi, L. (2020). *The XX Brain.* New York: Avery, 5.

7. Hölzel, B. K., Carmody, J., Vangel, M., Congleton, C., Yerramsetti, S. M., Gard, T., & Lazar, S. W. (2011). Mindfulness practice leads to increases in regional brain gray matter density. *Psychiatry Research, 191*(1), 36–43. https://doi.org/10.1016/j.pscychresns.2010.08.006.

8. Ke, S., Guimond, A., Tworoger, S., Huang, T., Chan, A., Liu, Y., & Kubzansky, L. (2023). Gut feelings: Associations of emotions and emotion regulation with the gut microbiome in women. *Psychological Medicine,* 1–10. doi:10.1017/S0033291723000612.

9. Satizabal, C. L., Himali, J. J., Beiser, A. S., Ramachandran, V., Melo van Lent, D., Himali, D., Aparicio, H. J., Maillard, P., DeCarli, C. S., Harris, W., & Seshadri, S. (2023). Association of red blood cell omega-3 fatty acids with MRI markers and cognitive function in midlife: The Framingham Heart Study. *Neurology, 99*(23), e2572–e2582. https://doi.org/10.1212/WNL.0000000000201296; Su, K., Tseng, P., Lin, P., et al. (2018). Association of use of omega-3 polyunsaturated fatty acids with changes in severity of anxiety symptoms: A systematic review and meta-analysis. *JAMA Network Open, 1*(5), e182327. doi:10.1001/jamanetworkopen.2018.2327; Yassine, H. N., Feng, Q., Azizkhanian, I., et al. (2016). Association of serum docosahexaenoic acid with cerebral amyloidosis. *JAMA Neurology, 73*(10), 1208–1216. doi:10.1001/jamaneurol.2016.1924.

10. Brody, B. (2022, July 18). What are nootropics? WebMD. https://www.webmd.com/vitamins-and-supplements/features/nootropics-smart-drugs-overview.

11. Salve, J., Pate, S., Debnath, K., & Langade, D. (2019). Adaptogenic and anxiolytic effects of ashwagandha root extract in healthy adults: A double-blind, randomized, placebo-controlled clinical study. *Cureus, 11*(12), e6466.

12. Levy, B. R. (2001). Eradication of ageism requires addressing the enemy within. *The Gerontologist, 41*(5), 578–580. https://doi.org/10.1093/geront/41.5.578.

13. Thomas, K. (2022). Safety first: Potential heart health risks of microdosing. Bill of Health (Harvard Law Petrie-Flom Center). https://blog.petrieflom.law.harvard.edu/2022/04/13/safety-first-potential-heart-health-risks-of-microdosing/; Winstock, A. R., Maier, L. J., Zhuparris, A., Davies, E., Puljevic, C., Kuypers, K. P. C., Ferris, J. A., & Barratt, M. J. (2021). Global drug survey (GDS) 2021 key findings report. https://www.globaldrugsurvey.com/wp-content/uploads/2021/12/Report2021_global.pdf; Carhart-Harris, R., Giribaldi, B., Watts, R., Baker-Jones, M., Murphy-Beiner, A., Murphy, R., Martell, J., Blemings, A., Erritzoe, D., & Nutt, D. J. (2021). Trial of psilocybin versus escitalopram for depression. *New England Journal of Medicine, 384*(15), 1402–1411; Shao, L.-X., Liao, C., Gregg, I., Davoudian, P. A., Savalia, N. K., Delagarza, K., & Kwan, A. C. (2021). Psilocybin induces rapid and persistent growth of dendritic spines in frontal cortex in vivo. *Neuron, 109*(16), 2535–2544.

14. Hutten, N. R. P. W., Mason, N. L., Dolder, P. C., Theunissen, E. L., Holze, F., Liechti, M. E., Varghese, N., Eckert, A., Feilding, A., Ramaekers, J. G., & Kuypers, K. P. C. (2021). Low doses of LSD acutely increase BDNF blood plasma levels in healthy volunteers. *ACS Pharmacology & Translational Science, 4*(2), 461–466. https://doi.org/10.1021/acsptsci.0c00099.

15. Bremner, J. D., Gurel, N. Z., Wittbrodt, M. T., Shandhi, M. H., Rapaport, M. H., Nye, J. A., Pearce, B. D., et al. (2020). Application of noninvasive vagal nerve stimulation to stress-related psychiatric disorders. *Journal of Personalized Medicine, 10*(3), 119; Tynan, A., Brines, M., & Chavan, S. S. (2022). Control of inflammation using non-invasive neuromodulation: Past, present and promise. *International Immunology, 34*(2), 119–128.

16. Salehpour, F., Khademi, M., Bragin, D. E., & DiDuro, J. O. (2022). Photobiomodulation therapy and the glymphatic system: Promising applications for augmenting the brain lymphatic drainage system. *International Journal of Molecular Sciences, 23*(6), 2975. https://doi.org/10.3390/ijms23062975.

17. Hamblin, M. R. (2016). Shining light on the head: Photobiomodulation for brain disorders. *BBA Clinical, 6,* 113–124. https://doi.org/10.1016/j.bbacli.2016.09.002.

18. Naeser, M. A., Zafonte, R., Krengel, M. H., Martin, P. I., Frazier, J., Hamblin, M. R., Knight, J. A., Meehan, W. P., III, & Baker, E. H. (2014). Significant improvements in cognitive performance post-transcranial, red/near-infrared light-emitting diode treatments in chronic, mild traumatic brain injury: Open-protocol study. *Journal of Neurotrauma, 31*(11), 1008–1017. https://doi.org/10.1089/neu.2013.3244; Figueiro Longo, M. G., Tan, C. O., Chan, S., et al. (2020). Effect of transcranial low-level light therapy vs sham therapy among patients with moderate traumatic brain injury: A randomized clinical trial. *JAMA Network Open, 3*(9), e2017337. doi:10.1001/jamanetworkopen.2020.17337.

19. Luo, G., Zhang, J., Song, Z., Wang, Y., Wang, X., Qu, H., Wang, F., Liu, C., & Gao, F. (2023). Effectiveness of non-pharmacological therapies on cognitive function in patients with dementia—a network meta-analysis of randomized controlled trials. *Frontiers in Aging Neuroscience, 15,* 1131744. https://doi.org/10.3389/fnagi.2023.1131744.

20. Enengl, J., Hamblin, M. R., & Dungel, P. (2020). Photobiomodulation for Alzheimer's disease: Translating basic research to clinical application. *Journal of Alzheimer's Disease, 75*(4), 1073–1082. https://doi.org/10.3233/JAD-191210.

21. Chan, D., Suk, H.-J., Jackson, B. L., Milman, N. P., Stark, D., Klerman, E. B., Kitchener, E., et al. (2022). Gamma frequency sensory stimulation in mild probable Alzheimer's dementia patients: Results of feasibility and pilot studies. *PloS ONE, 17*(12), e0278412.

22. Sachdeva, S., Persaud, S., Patel, M., Popard, P., Colverson, A., & Doré, S. (2022). Effects of sound interventions on the permeability of the blood-brain barrier and meningeal lymphatic clearance. *Brain Sciences, 12*(6), 742. https://doi.org/10.3390/brainsci12060742.

23. Aleksijević, L. H., Aleksijević, M., Škrlec, I., Šram, M., Šram, M., & Talapko, J. (2022). *Porphyromonas gingivalis* virulence factors and clinical significance in periodontal disease and coronary artery diseases. *Pathogens, 11*(10), 1173. https://doi.org/10.3390/pathogens11101173.

24. Lehrer, S., & Rheinstein, P. H. (2022). Vaccination reduces risk of Alzheimer's disease, Parkinson's disease and other neurodegenerative disorders. *Discovery Medicine, 34*(172), 97–101.

25. Pereira Oliva, H. N., Mansur Machado, F. S., Rodrigues, V. D., Leão, L. L., & Monteiro-Júnior, R. S. (2020). The effect of dual-task training on cognition of

people with different clinical conditions: An overview of systematic reviews. *IBRO Reports, 9*, 24–31. https://doi.org/10.1016/j.ibror.2020.06.005.

26. Mosconi, *The XX Brain*, 196.
27. Gentreau, M., Chuy, V., Féart, C., Samieri, C., Ritchie, K., Raymond, M., Berticat, C., & Artero, S. (2020). Refined carbohydrate-rich diet is associated with long-term risk of dementia and Alzheimer's disease in apolipoprotein E ε4 allele carriers. *Alzheimer's & Dementia: The Journal of the Alzheimer's Association, 16*(7), 1043–1053. https://doi.org/10.1002/alz.12114.
28. Pereira Oliva, et al. The effect of dual-task training on cognition of people with different clinical conditions.
29. Mosconi, *The XX Brain*, 197.
30. Boere, K., Lloyd, K., Binsted, G., & Krigolosin, O. E. (2023). Exercising is good for the brain but exercising outside is potentially better. *Scientific Reports, 13*, 1140. https://doi.org/10.1038/s41598-022-26093-2.
31. Dominy, S. S., Lynch, C., Ermini, F., Benedyk, M., Marczyk, A., Konradi, A., Nguyen, M., Haditsch, U., Raha, D., Griffin, C., Holsinger, L. J., Arastu-Kapur, S., Kaba, S., Lee, A., Ryder, M. I., Potempa, B., Mydel, P., Hellvard, A., Adamowicz, K., Hasturk, H., et al. (2019). *Porphyromonas gingivalis* in Alzheimer's disease brains: Evidence for disease causation and treatment with small-molecule inhibitors. *Science Advances, 5*(1), eaau3333. https://doi.org/10.1126/sciadv.aau3333.
32. Nadim, R., Tang, J., Dilmohamed, A., Yuan, S., Wu, C., Bakre, A. T., Partridge, M., Ni, J., Copeland, J. R., Anstey, K. J., & Chen, R. (2020). Influence of periodontal disease on risk of dementia: A systematic literature review and a meta-analysis. *European Journal of Epidemiology, 35*(9), 821–833. https://doi.org/10.1007/s10654-020-00648-x.

CHAPTER 10

1. Holt-Lunstad, J., Smith, T. B., Baker, M., Harris, T., & Stephenson, D. (2015). Loneliness and social isolation as risk factors for mortality: A meta-analytic review. *Perspectives on Psychological Science, 10*(2), 227–237.
2. National Academies of Sciences, Engineering, and Medicine. (2020). *Social isolation and loneliness in older adults: Opportunities for the health care system.* Washington, DC: National Academies Press.
3. Wizemann, T., ed. (2015). *Business engagement in building healthy communities: Workshop summary.* Washington, DC: National Academies Press.
4. Mineo, L. (2017, April 11). Good genes are nice, but joy is better. *Harvard Gazette.* https://news.harvard.edu/gazette/story/2017/04/over-nearly-80-years-harvard-study-has-been-showing-how-to-live-a-healthy-and-happy-life/.
5. Administration on Aging. (2022). 2021 Profile of Older Americans. Administration for Community Living, U.S. Department of Health and Human Services. https://acl.gov/sites/default/files/Profile%20of%20OA/2021%20Profile%20of%20OA/2021ProfileOlderAmericans_508.pdf.
6. McCraty, R., Barrios-Choplin, B., Rozman, D., Atkinson, M., & Watkins, A. D. (1998). The impact of a new emotional self-management program on stress, emotions, heart rate variability, DHEA and cortisol. *Integrative*

Physiological and Behavioral Science: The Official Journal of the Pavlovian Society, 33(2), 151–170. https://doi.org/10.1007/BF02688660.

7. Whillans, A., Dunn, E., Sandstrom, G., Dickerson, S., & Madden, K. (2015). Is spending money on others good for your heart? *Health Psychology: Official Journal of the Division of Health Psychology, American Psychological Association, 35*(6), 574–583. https://doi.org/10.1037/hea0000332.

8. Brown, S. L., Nesse, R. M., Vinokur, A. D., & Smith, D. M. (2003). Providing social support may be more beneficial than receiving it: Results from a prospective study of mortality. *Psychological Science, 14*(4), 320–327.

9. Hui, B. P. H., Ng, J. C. K., Berzaghi, E. Cunningham-Amos, L. A., & Kogan, A. (2020). Rewards of kindness? A meta-analysis of the link between prosociality and well-being. *Psychological Bulletin, 146* (12), 1084–1116. https://doi.org/10.1037/bul0000298.

10. Edward Jones and Age Wave. (2023). Resilient choices: Trade-offs, adjustments, and course corrections to thrive in retirement. https://www.edwardjones.com/sites/default/files/acquiadam/2023-05/050423_AW_EJ_4Pillar_ResilientChoices_FINAL.pdf.

11. Alimujiang, A., Wiensch, A., Boss, J., Fleischer, N. L., Mondul, A. M., McLean, K., Mukherjee, B., & Pearce, C. L. (2019). Association between life purpose and mortality among US adults older than 50 years. *JAMA Network Open, 2*(5), e194270.

12. Edward Jones, Age Wave, and the Harris Poll. (2021). The four pillars of the new retirement: Tracking update with a spotlight on family.

13. Irving, J., Davis, S., & Collier, A. (2017). Aging with purpose: Systematic search and review of literature pertaining to older adults and purpose. *International Journal of Aging & Human Development, 85*(4), 403–437. https://doi.org/10.1177/0091415017702908.

14. Sonnega, A. (2017). The Health and Retirement Study: Aging in the 21st century, challenges and opportunities for Americans. Survey Research Center, Institute for Social Research, University of Michigan. https://hrsonline.isr.umich.edu/sitedocs/databook/inc/pdf/HRS-Aging-in-the-21St-Century.pdf.

CHAPTER 11

1. Hanson, M. (2021, December 16). Student loan debt by gender. EducationData.org. https://educationdata.org/student-loan-debt-by-gender.

2. Age Wave estimate based on U.S. Bureau of Labor Statistics, Number of jobs, labor market experience, and earnings growth: Results from a national longitudinal survey, 2017. https://www.bls.gov/news.release/archives/nlsoy_08242017.htm.

3. James, J. (2022). How America saves. Vanguard. https://institutional.vanguard.com/content/dam/inst/vanguard-has/insights-pdfs/22_TL_HAS_FullReport_2022.pdf.

4. King, B. (2022). Those who married once more likely than others to have retirement savings. United States Census Bureau. https://www.census.gov/library/stories/2022/01/women-more-likely-than-men-to-have-no-retirement-savings.html.

5. Aragão, C. (2023.) Gender pay gap in U.S. hasn't changed much in two decades. https://www.pewresearch.org/short-reads/2023/03/01/gender-pay-gap-facts/.

6. Center for American Progress (2023). What to know about the gender wage gap as the equal pay act turns 60. https://www.americanprogress.org/article/what-to-know-about-the-gender-wage-gap-as-the-equal-pay-act-turns-60.

7. Wilson, C. (2019). Just how bad is the gender pay gap? Brutal, when you look at a lifetime of work. *Time.* https://time.com/5562269/equal-pay-day-women-men-lifetime-wages/.

8. Fox, M. (2021). As interest in investing grows, people of color still lag behind, CNBC survey finds. CNBC. https://www.cnbc.com/2021/08/23/as-interest-in-investing-grows-people-of-color-still-lag-behind-cnbc-survey-finds.html.

9. Hernández Kent, A. (2021). Gender wealth gaps in the U.S. and the benefits of closing them. Federal Reserve Bank of St. Louis. https://www.stlouisfed.org/en/open-vault/2021/september/gender-wealth-gaps-us-benefits-of-closing-them.

10. Fidelity Investments. (2021). Women and Investing Study. https://www.fidelity.com/bin-public/060_www_fidelity_com/documents/about-fidelity/FidelityInvestmentsWomen&InvestingStudy2021.pdf.

11. Barber, B. M., & Odean, T. (2001). Boys will be boys: Gender, overconfidence, and common stock investment. *Quarterly Journal of Economics.* https://faculty.haas.berkeley.edu/odean/papers/gender/boyswillbeboys.pdf.

12. Huang, J., & DeLuca, T. J. (2020). The same but different: Gender and investor behavior. Vanguard Research. https://static.vgcontent.info/crp/intl/avw/mexico/documents/gender-and-investor-behavior.pdf.

13. Lieber, R. (2021, October 29). Women may be better investors than men. Let me mansplain why. *New York Times.* https://www.nytimes.com/2021/10/29/your-money/women-investing-stocks.html.

14. Nationwide. (2022). Women investors pivot to more proactive approach in financial planning. https://news.nationwide.com/030322-women-investors-more-proactive-financial-planning/.

15. Fidelity Investments. Women and Investing Study.

16. Gillespie, L. (2023). Survey: 69% have made a financial sacrifice to help their adult children with money. Bankrate. https://www.bankrate.com/personal-finance/financial-independence-survey/.

17. Merrill Lynch and Age Wave. (2018). Women & financial wellness: Beyond the bottom line.

18. Fry, R., Aragão, C., Hurst, K., & Parker, K. (2023.) In a growing share of U.S. marriages, husbands and wives earn about the same. Pew Research Center. https://www.pewresearch.org/social-trends/2023/04/13/in-a-growing-share-of-u-s-marriages-husbands-and-wives-earn-about-the-same/.

19. Bongai, P., Howard, O., Prakash, L., & Zucker, J. (2020). Women as the next wave of growth in wealth management. McKinsey. https://www.mckinsey.com/industries/financial-services/our-insights/women-as-the-next-wave-of-growth-in-us-wealth-management.

20. CPI Inflation Calculator. U.S. Bureau of Labor Statistics. https://www.bls.gov/data/inflation_calculator.htm.

21. Woold, S. H., Aron, L., Dubay, L., Simon, S. M., Zimmerman, E., & Luk, K. X. (2015). How are income and wealth linked to health and longevity? https://www.aspeninstitute.org/wp-content/uploads/2017/03/Urban-Institute -How-Are-Income-and-Wealth-Linked.pdf.

22. Yamamoto, D. H. (2013). Health care costs—from birth to death. Health Care Cost Institute Report.

23. National Association of Insurance Commissioners (revised 2019). A shopper's guide to long-term care insurance. https://content.naic.org/sites/default/files /publication-ltc-lp-shoppers-guide-long-term.pdf.

24. Global Impact Investing Network. (n.d.). What you need to know about impact investing. Retrieved July 5, 2023, from https://thegiin.org/impact -investing/need-to-know/.

25. Edward Jones and Age Wave. (2021). The four pillars of the new retirement: What a difference a year makes. https://www.edwardjones.com/sites/default /files/acquiadam/2021-06/Four-Pillars-US-Report-June-2021.pdf.

INDEX